Beat
Back Pain

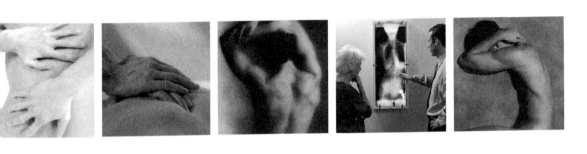

52 Brilliant Ideas

one good idea can change your life

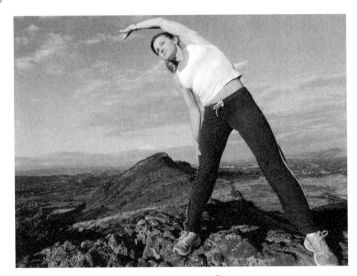

Beat Back Pain

Smart and Simple Ways to Ease the Strain

Ruth Chambers, MD

A Perigee Book

A PERIGEE BOOK
Published by the Penguin Group
Penguin Group (USA) Inc.
375 Hudson Street, New York, New York 10014, USA
Penguin Group (Canada), 90 Eglinton Avenue East, Suite 700, Toronto, Ontario M4P 2Y3, Canada
(a division of Pearson Penguin Canada Inc.)
Penguin Books Ltd., 80 Strand, London WC2R 0RL, England
Penguin Group Ireland, 25 St. Stephen's Green, Dublin 2, Ireland (a division of Penguin Books Ltd.)
Penguin Group (Australia), 250 Camberwell Road, Camberwell, Victoria 3124, Australia
(a division of Pearson Australia Group Pty. Ltd.)
Penguin Books India Pvt. Ltd., 11 Community Centre, Panchsheel Park, New Delhi—110 017, India
Penguin Group (NZ), 67 Apollo Drive, Rosedale, North Shore 0632, New Zealand
(a division of Pearson New Zealand Ltd.)
Penguin Books (South Africa) (Pty.) Ltd., 24 Sturdee Avenue, Rosebank, Johannesburg 2196,
South Africa

Penguin Books Ltd., Registered Offices: 80 Strand, London WC2R 0RL, England

While the author has made every effort to provide accurate telephone numbers and Internet addresses at the time of publication, neither the publisher nor the author assumes any responsibility for errors, or for changes that occur after publication. Further, the publisher does not have any control over and does not assume any responsibility for author or third-party websites or their content.

BEAT BACK PAIN

First American edition: June 2008
Originally published in Great Britain in 2005 by The Infinite Ideas Company Limited.

Perigee trade paperback ISBN: 978-0-399-53389-1

PRINTED IN THE UNITED STATES OF AMERICA

10   9   8   7   6   5   4   3   2   1

PUBLISHER'S NOTE: Neither the publisher nor the author is engaged in rendering professional advice or services to the individual reader. The ideas, procedures, and suggestions contained in this book are not intended as a substitute for consulting with your physician. All matters regarding your health require medical supervision. Neither the author nor the publisher shall be liable or responsible for any loss or damage allegedly arising from any information or suggestion in this book.

Most Perigee books are available at special quantity discounts for bulk purchases for sales promotions, premiums, fund-raising, or educational use. Special books, or book excerpts, can also be created to fit specific needs. For details, write: Special Markets, Penguin Group (USA) Inc., 375 Hudson Street, New York, New York 10014.

Brilliant ideas

Brilliant features

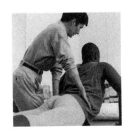

Each chapter of this book is designed to provide you with an inspirational idea that you can read quickly and put into practice right away.

Throughout you'll find four features that will help you to get right to the heart of the idea:

- *Try another idea* If this idea looks like a life-changer then there's no time to lose. *Try another idea* will point you right to a related tip to expand and enhance the first.

- *Here's an idea for you* Give it a try—right here, right now—and get an idea of how well you're doing so far.

- *Defining ideas* Words of wisdom from masters and mistresses of the art, plus some interesting, hangers-on.

- *How did it go?* If at first you do succeed, try to hide your amazement. If, on the other hand, you don't this is where you'll find a Q and A that highlights common problems and how to get over them.

Introduction

Miserable, isn't it? Something as simple as back pain standing between you and a normal life.

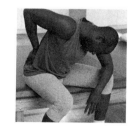

Can't play with young kids, can't travel long distances, can't do the chores (ah, shame!), can't have sex when and where you want to (have you ever?). So you've got to get back your life, control your pain, obliterate that stiffness. And here's how you do it. Read through this book to savor each individual idea. All are different, and any or all could be your lifesavers. Go on, try some out. When you find one that works well, you can do it again and again and again...though maybe you won't need to if it gets your back right.

There are heart transplants, kidney transplants, even hair transplants—but they don't do back transplants (yet), so it's up to you to make your back last a lifetime. That's about building up your muscles to keep your spine strong, just to cope with everyday living. Easier said than done, as you'll have to make new life resolutions to keep fit—and stay fit forever, no letting up. So get ready for a full-on back makeover.

In this book you'll find ideas to help yourself. You'll come to realize that your world is a dangerous place. Squaring up to your computer, lightening the loads you lift, being straight with yourself—these are all ways you'll use your brain to prevent back strain. And it's not just thinking about how to keep your back safe you want to develop, it's positive thinking, too. Mind and matter. Many of the ideas here rely on you making the best of how your back is shaping up. Making the time for exercise and keeping fit rather than wishing you could turn the clock back to when you were younger and in ace condition.

There's no shortage of people out there waiting to help you, either: the sports therapist, the osteopath, the chiropractor, the doctor, the herbalist, the homeopath, the physical therapist, and more are all sitting there saying me, me, me! You'll get a good idea about how to use them and when. Bone up on what they offer, if you haven't had the nerve to consult them before. Reading up on how your spine moves will help you understand how their treatments work and why you should give them a try.

Conventional medicine doesn't have all the answers. It has some—and pain-killing drugs or even surgery might be just what you need at a certain time. But fortunately there are lots of alternatives, and trying these out should help you to avoid taking drugs. *Roll a joint* in this book means learning to do Pilates exercises, finding out more about the massage you'll be kneading, or taking your therapist's manipulation lying down. *Popping a pill* could be one from the herbalist or homeopath, or one that you buy over the counter—not necessarily a prescription from your doctor.

Believe it or not, this book will also save you money—lots of money. First, by getting your back in shape and keeping it that way, you won't lose so much time off work. Second, there are lots of ideas here for you to try to help yourself, so you're less likely to need costly therapy. And if you do need to consult a therapist or doctor, armed with the knowledge gleaned from these pages, you'll be more likely to choose the right one for your back problem immediately.

If you've got back pain and don't know where to turn, try turning the pages of this book to set you on your way—lots of ways, in fact. You're bound to have more questions when you've tried out an idea—and funnily enough, we've given you a lot of the answers, too! Almost all aspects of your life are touched on in this book. Whether it's moving, digging in the garden, going on vacation, doing your hobbies, having a baby, or driving your car—there's a backlog of solutions here.

One last thing: Make sure you're sitting comfortably when you read the book—skip to IDEA 4 and check out your posture. There, you're off, you've started already...

1
Lesson 1–it's in the works

Bone up on your anatomy and you'll understand more about how your spine works. Flex your muscles and stretch those ligaments–within limits.

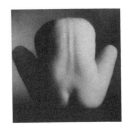

Discover how to stand, move, and live more comfortably.

IT'S NOT UNUSUAL

You're not miserable alone. More than two-thirds of people get low back pain at some time in their lives. It's most common in 35- to 55-year-olds. About 1 in 12 adults goes to see their family doctor about their back pain in any one year. It's funny, but when you have back pain everyone has a story to tell you about theirs, too.

HOW DOES YOUR SPINE WORK?

Let's get the difficult stuff over with. Your spine is a column of thirty-three bones, the vertebrae. These form the basic structure of the spine. The vertebrae are stacked neatly on top of one another like interlocking bricks. You have seven cervical vertebrae in your neck, with the top one linking to your skull, twelve thoracic vertebrae in your chest, five large lumbar vertebrae in your middle or lower back, five sacral vertebrae in your low back, linking your spine to your pelvic girdle, and four bones in your coccyx.

Information is power. As you understand more about how your back works, you'll be able to figure out what to do to avoid straining it and help it to get better. Visualize the effect when your facet joints swell up: You'll get pain and your back might lock. If it does, you can see you'll need to move about as much as possible to prevent your spine from seizing up. Imagine what happens when you build up the muscles running alongside your spine: You'll strengthen the support for your spinal column and be able to resist all sorts of pressures and trauma.

They join together in a series of curves that give your spine strength and flexibility. And wow, do you need that strength!

The vertebral bodies are the main load-bearing part of your spine. Muscles and ligaments are attached, too. The ligaments are tough fibers that are there to keep everything in place. Bony arches extend from the back of the vertebrae to form the spinal canal. This is a sort of protective tunnel running the length of your spine and down where nerves pass from your brain to the rest of your body. Nerves emerge from gaps between each pair of bones to supply your muscles and carry sensation to your brain. The nerves to the legs emerge from the lumbar-sacral part of the spine. Some of these join to make up the bundle of nerve fibers known as the sciatic nerve, which supplies the leg and foot.

Between the bones are the intervertebral discs, which cushion your spine from jarring and enable it to move even when you're carrying a weight. The intervertebral discs make up about a quarter of the height of the spine. Discs come in two parts: a central jelly, which supports the weight, and a series of concentric rings, which keep the jelly in place. Behind the disc is a notch through which the nerve passes, and behind this is a "facet" joint, which allows one bone to move on another. All the bones are joined together by ligaments.

Major muscle groups also support and stabilize the spine. These are responsible for providing the spine with the power to flex, extend, twist, and bend sideways.

And so ends today's lesson on anatomy.

Being under stress can increase the pain you get from muscle spasm. So try IDEA 27, *Stress buster*, to find ways to put you in control.

Try another idea...

WHAT IS BACK PAIN?

Most back pain comes from the muscles, ligaments, and joints in your back. When and where you get back pain depends on what the cause is, whether the pain arises from the spine, ligaments, and muscles around it, or whether a nerve is trapped at its root, which can cause pain along its length, like sciatica.

"Lower back pain" is what you feel in the small of your back. "Acute" lasts for six weeks or less; if it lasts longer than that, it's "chronic"—ouch! Unfortunately, it's common for back pain to recur over the years.

HOW ARE YOU DOING?

As you get older, the water content of your intervertebral discs decreases, causing the discs to narrow. They become less able to stand up to wear and tear and are more easily damaged. If they don't hold the vertebrae far enough apart, the nerves may be squashed where they emerge from your spine, causing you pain, numbness, or pins and needles. Your spine also becomes less flexible as you grow older and is more likely to be strained.

"All we actually have is our body and its muscles that allow us to be under our own power."
ALLEGRA KENT, ballerina

Defining idea...

3

Occasionally a nerve can become trapped by part of the disc between the bones of the spine oozing out and squashing it. Being in a bent-forward posture for a long time or lifting with a bent back can cause the central jelly of the disc to move backward as pressure is put on the front of the disc. This type of problem usually gets better on its own as the jelly gets sucked back into place when the pressure is removed.

How did it go? **Q** **My back is really causing me some pain. It can't be natural. I don't want to worry unnecessarily, but how do I know when my back pain is serious?**

A *If it's a simple backache, there's nothing to worry about. If there is no sign of any serious damage or underlying disease, you should have a full recovery in a few days or weeks. That means no permanent weakness.*

Q **I strained my back a whole week ago, and I'm still in agony. Should I get treatment immediately, or should I wait and see if it gets better?**

A *Low back pain usually gets better by itself—though I'm afraid it may take a little longer than a week. But you don't want to be one of the statistics that show that once a person has been out of work with back pain for six months they have about a one in two chance of ever returning to work. So do whatever it takes to beat your back pain—no need to consult your doctor yet, unless you think there are complications.*

2
Lesson 2–don't panic

It's simple, it's a slip or strain, your muscles are stiff, or a pinched nerve is causing your pain.

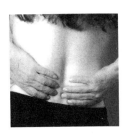

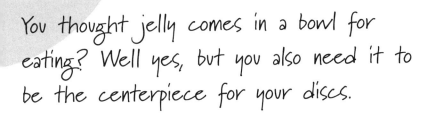

You thought jelly comes in a bowl for eating? Well yes, but you also need it to be the centerpiece for your discs.

PUT SIMPLY

Backache is labeled as "simple" if the pain is triggered by a mechanical source of some sort. Bang! You've got pain arising from the bony part of your spine or the muscles attached to it. And boy, is it painful! The pain may spread in a general way down to one or both of your hips, thighs, and legs. The difference between simple backache and other types of back pain is that your lumbar or sciatic nerve roots or the spinal cord are not compressed.

People who suffer from simple backache are usually between 20 and 55 years old, and are otherwise generally healthy. Their pain is in the small of their back, buttocks, and thighs. Their symptoms vary depending on what physical activities they're doing and the time of day (for example, they often get worse just before it's time to do the dishes).

Here's an idea for you...

Believe that you'll get better. Pain doesn't necessarily mean damage to your spine: most pain is due to a strain of the ligaments and muscles around your spine, and settles down fairly quickly. A slipped disc does usually get better by itself. So before investing in a bell so you can ring for service at home, remember that most people with back pain recover from an acute attack within 6 weeks.

SLIPPED DISC

A slipped disc can be caused by poor posture, a jarring accident, or lifting something incorrectly. The jelly-like center of the intervertebral disc can be forced through the outer rings of the disc because of the excessive vertical pressure on your spine. Putting more pressure on the front of a disc pushes the jelly backward (though sideways slippage of the jelly can sometimes occur). This can happen when you're sitting or standing for long periods with your lumbar spine flattened, instead of maintaining it with the correct curve. Lifting a weight by bending forward similarly puts strain on the front of the disc. The force causing the slipped disc may also damage ligaments of your spine, facet joints of your vertebrae, and nearby muscles.

The slipped disc then presses on your nerve roots as they emerge from your spinal canal, giving you pain and muscle spasm. You'll feel this as pain or pins and needles along the path of the particular nerve, which could be in your buttock, thigh, or foot.

Slipped discs are also known as herniated, ruptured, or prolapsed discs.

NERVE ROOT PAIN

A pinched nerve is usually caused by the prolapse or slipping of an intervertebral disc, narrowing the spinal canal where the nerves pass through, or from scarring caused by previous surgery. The pain from the pinched nerve root passes along the site that the nerve travels down, to the ending of that strand of nerve at your skin.

Sciatic pain follows the left or right branch of the sciatic nerve from your lumbar–sacral spine at the bottom of your back to shoot down to your thigh, knee, or foot on the same side of your body. This is sciatica. Sometimes you can lose sensation around the same area, get pins and needles or tingling, or your muscles become weaker. The ligaments in your spine may be damaged, too, or you may get muscle spasm, making your back feel stiff or even "locked," so that you can barely move.

Occasionally a slipped disc presses on the nerves supplying your bladder or bowel, making it difficult for you to urinate or pass feces. If this happens or you have severe weakness or numbness in one of your legs, get medical help immediately. See IDEA 33, *At the cutting edge*, to learn more about these red flags.

Try another idea...

SACRO-ILIAC STRAIN AND STIFFNESS

The ligaments or joints on each side of your sacrum can also be strained. Women are more prone to this during pregnancy, when their ligaments have become lax in readiness for giving birth. Gymnasts develop loose and supple joints, too. Your sacro-iliac joints can become inflamed in various conditions such as ankylosing spondylitis, which may involve all the vertebrae of your low back.

SOMETHING NASTY

It's rare, but back pain could be the first you know about an infection or a tumor. If a tumor does grow in your spine it has usually spread there from somewhere else in your body, and

"It is better to know some of the questions than all of the answers."
JAMES THURBER

Defining idea...

7

you'll probably have other symptoms, such as weight loss, loss of appetite, tiredness, and feeling unwell. Infections in the spine usually only occur in people who are susceptible to infection, such as people with diabetes, or those who misuse drugs or alcohol.

How did it go?

Q **How quickly should my backache improve? I don't want to push it, but I'm due to play golf next week.**

A *Most cases of severe back pain improve a lot in a few days, or at most a few weeks. Milder symptoms may last longer, and can often go on for a few months. Ninety percent recover within six weeks, but about one in twelve people develop chronic pain that lasts longer. Are you feeling lucky?*

Q **Once I'm over a nasty bout of back pain, how can I be sure it won't come back?**

A *"Sure" and "won't" are such strong words! You might think you've gotten over your back pain and it's all in the past, but then unluckily something happens—an awkward lift, an unexpected sneeze—and you're struck with pain again. Watch out, because when people have pain, they often adopt certain postures that relieve their pain temporarily but cause even more problems in the long term. Their ligaments and muscles shorten or lengthen to adapt to their new, perhaps slumped, posture. Then minor backache can develop into a long-standing problem. But don't despair, you can take measures to minimize the risks.*

3

Help yourself

Go ahead, help yourself. Not to just anything, but to better health and no back pain. So take as many helpings of exercise and sensible living as you want.

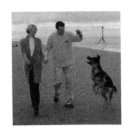

To minimize your back pain, use your brain.
Go for a walk or start to train.

STAY ACTIVE

Most backaches aren't serious, even if it feels that way. You might have to take things easy for a day or so, but don't play the invalid and take to your bed—resting will do you more harm than good. You'll get more stiff and develop muscle degeneration of your back and other joints. And you'll lose Brownie points with whoever it is running around tending to your every need.

Lying in bed, you'll think more about the pain and may get depressed. The longer you lie there, the harder it'll be to get going again. You might even get bedsores, and if you're really unlucky you could develop a clot or deep venous thrombosis. Next thing you know, you'll have a heart attack or stroke—and then try getting out of bed! So get up and about, even if you need to take painkillers to do so.

Even if you can't do all your normal activities at first, you can do some. Go for a walk. Keeping as active and normal as possible will help your recovery. You'll feel healthier, use less painkillers, and be less distressed by your pain.

Here's an idea for you... **Buy a back stretcher and lie on it for 10 minutes a day. It's an arch shape, made of wood, and has many knobs on it. When you lie on the knobs, the muscles running alongside your spine take your weight. This helps to keep your spine in its natural position. You can even do exercises while you're lying on the back stretcher.**

BOOST YOUR PHYSICAL HEALTH AND GENERAL WELL-BEING

They say prevention is better than cure (whoever they are), and they're right. People often hurt their backs by doing sudden unaccustomed exercise, like intensive gardening or home repairs. So avoid the problem by increasing your fitness and building up your muscles. Regular exercise will also make you feel good by releasing natural chemicals which'll lift your mood and reduce your pain.

Try a lifestyle makeover. Stop smoking—people who smoke are more likely to suffer from back pain than non-smokers. All that coughing can jar the spine, too. Get that excess weight off and keep it off. It's only adding extra stress to your spine.

Defining idea... *"Always bear in mind that your own resolution to succeed is more important than any one thing."* ABRAHAM LINCOLN

A POSITIVE ATTITUDE SAYS IT ALL

By not dwelling on your ill health or disability you'll minimize the effects of your back pain and any other illnesses. Think positive. Remember that you're likely to improve within a few days. Distract yourself by reading, listening to music, or chatting with your friends.

Get on with your life despite the pain. The more you enjoy life and are interested in your work, the less important your backache will seem. Avoid taking time off work if possible. You don't have to wait until you're pain-free to start work unless you're in a heavily physical job. Focus on returning to work as quickly as possible.

See IDEA 34, *Moving forward*, for more insights on keeping a positive mental attitude and making the most of things, despite your back problems.

Try another idea...

REMEMBER HOW TO LIFT

Stay alert! Constantly be aware of how you're lifting heavy or awkward loads. Don't just shove that bed back against the wall: Think about what you're doing and move it correctly. Don't lift that pile of papers off the seat to oblige someone without considering the best way to do it. If they want to sit down, let them lift it!

STRAIGHT UP

Stand straight. Slouching forward, as most of us tend to do, stretches the ligaments of your back, especially if you're overweight. Go for flatter, broad-heeled shoes. When you sit try to remain upright with a slight hollow in your back. If you are a natural slumper, put a small cushion or rolled-up towel in the hollow of your back for extra support. Always be aware of how you sit and stand.

"Rise, take up thy bed, and walk."
THE GOSPEL, according to St. John

Defining idea...

11

SEE A DOCTOR

Before seeking medical advice, try simple painkillers or ice or heat therapy. But if your pain gets worse or spreads, or other complications set in, get medical help as soon as possible. If you've had a bad fall and are lying in agony from your back, don't move and ask someone else to summon help in case you've fractured your back or other limbs. (And try not to land on your cell phone—you may need it!) The medics visiting you at the scene can make sure that any movement you make doesn't do any more damage than you've done already.

How did it go?

Q   **When my back hurts it's difficult to be active—should I take painkillers then, so I can get out and about?**

A   *In a word—yes, unless you can control your pain by other means. Moving around is good for you. And remember, if you have a simple backache you're not causing damage to your back by keeping active. Stop doing an activity, though, if it makes your back worse.*

Q   **I'm a competitive person and tend to push myself to the limit. Should I avoid playing sports when I have back pain in case I damage my back by overdoing it?**

A   *This may be difficult for you, but try to be rational. Some exercises, like swimming, walking, and cycling, are easier to do than others when you've got a bad back. You're more in control in these types of sports, and you can stop for rests at will. And they're not going to encourage your competitive streak. If you try a more challenging sport but find a particular movement is agony, then don't do it! You'll get your chance later, when your back has recovered.*

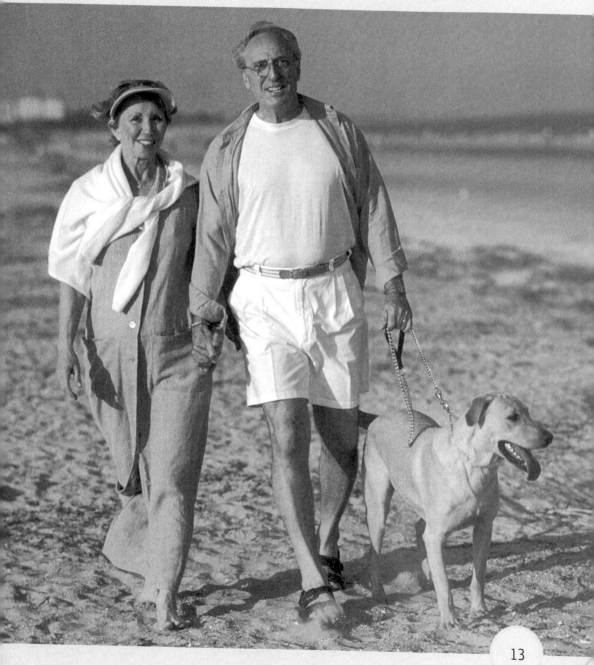

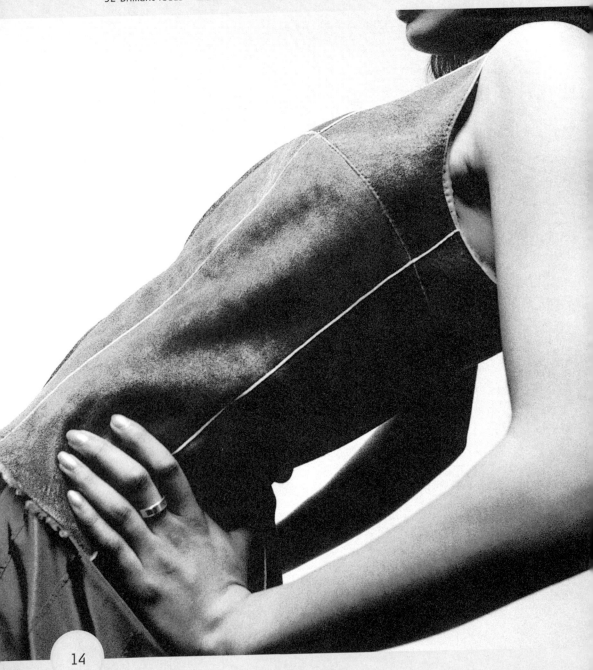

4

Hold your head up high

Imagine you're on the catwalk, gliding along, head up, back straight, tail in. All right, it's a pretty tall order—but you can still do the head-up/straight-back part.

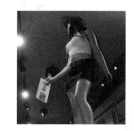

Position yourself to succeed. Never slouch when you can sit, or sit slumped when you can lie, or lie crooked when you can be at all times well-supported.

ALL THE TIME

Think about your posture all day, every day. Anyone who crouches in cramped positions at work will eventually get a bad back. Look at Quasimodo—if he hasn't spent all day, every day hunched over a computer I don't know who has! Take regular breaks or stretch out frequently if you're doing repetitive movements or sitting or standing still for long periods.

When the natural curves of your spine are preserved, there is less compression of your intervertebral discs and less strain on your back ligaments. And it's not just the position of your back you should think of. When all your other joints are well positioned then the strain on your back ligaments and tendons is minimal.

To lie comfortably opt for a fairly firm mattress with your head and neck supported so that your spine remains as straight as possible. If the mattress is too soft or sags, you will sink into it and your spine will curve unnaturally; too hard, and your spine will be an unsupported bridge between your shoulders and hips.

POOR POSTURE

Sitting can cause your pelvis to rotate backward, causing your lumbar spine to bend with it. This then compresses your intervertebral discs and the cartilage between. Raising your arms in front of your body (for instance, typing on a keyboard) or lifting objects while sitting in this position increases the pressure even more. The damage is worse if the muscles around your spine holding you in position become tired.

Being overweight or obese will pull your spine into an unnatural position that makes it more susceptible to wear and tear and may perpetuate your back pain. So if you're tubby, do something about it.

Sleeping on your stomach can put extra strain on your neck. If there's some reason preventing you from lying flat, you may need to adapt your posture, perhaps by raising the top end of your bed by 4–5 inches. Some people who suffer from back pain have found that a waterbed helps, others say that it makes their waves of pain worse.

SITTING POSITION

A firm, high-backed chair is ideal. Sitting upright, well back on the chair with a lumbar roll or small cushion in your lower back will give your lumbar spine support and make you look very important. Find a chair that supports your head and neck if possible. Avoid low chairs, or sitting with your legs straight out in front of you on the floor or in bed, as it puts strain on the base of your back. Don't curl up in an armchair with your legs tucked underneath you either, as your spine will be forced into a sharp curve.

Play music when you're sitting around. Unconsciously fidgeting in time to the music will keep you gently active without thinking about it.

Choose a car that not only fulfills your driving needs but is also just right for your back. One with widely adjustable driving positions will enable you to get comfortable. See IDEA 42, *Driving force*, for other clues on taking the pain out of driving.

Try another idea...

LET'S NOT TWIST AGAIN

Okay, it's difficult to remember, but try to keep upright, and maintain the curves of your lumbar spine and neck. Don't slouch—pretend that someone from a modeling agency might be out there spotting you (and that you've always wanted to be a model). If your lower back becomes flatter, you'll become round-shouldered and your chin will poke forward. Walk around with your head held high and shoulders down, swinging your arms gently.

When standing, try to place equal weight on each foot, especially if you're in one position for a long time. If you have a standing job, make sure the height of your working surface is comfortable. Rather than reach or stretch too far while standing in one place, move nearer to the object you're working with if possible. Avoid twisting from your waist by moving your feet instead.

Many everyday activities, such as ironing, vacuum cleaning, watching TV, and shopping, can cause problems if you do them with poor posture. Try to do them in ways that avoid putting excess strain on your spine.

"Never grow a wishbone...where your backbone ought to be."
CLEMENTINE PADDLEFORD, food editor

Defining idea...

17

You need to watch your back particularly when gardening. Bend your knees and not your back when you're digging and weeding. Kneel down when you're planting, so you can keep your back straight instead of bending over.

How did it go?

Q   So all I have to do is remember to stand or sit all the time. Do you realize I have the attention span of a gnat? What else can I do to improve my posture?

A   *If you study Pilates you'll learn some excellent exercises to strengthen your muscles, especially the ones that maintain your trunk in a good position. That'll include your abdominal muscles and back muscles, which you'll be able to use to control the shape of your spine. You could also try the Alexander Technique to learn the correct ways to stand and sit, and to improve your posture. Where your head leads, your spine follows.*

Q   It's great to discuss how to sit with good posture, but I have to stand for my job. Can I do anything to help myself?

A   *You should bend over backward to help yourself. By doing backward bends, you will vary your position and temporarily relieve all the stresses and strains that have built up with your normal position. Try doing them every 20 minutes or so. Back flips are optional.*

5

Ergonomics—pure science

**It sounds complicated, but it's a simple equation:
your comfort + health + productivity = ergonomics.**

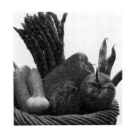

We're talking round pegs in round holes,
not square pegs in any old shaped holes,
slats, pits, or slight indentations.

PUT YOURSELF FIRST

Ergonomics is a science. Not the white coats and animal rights demonstrations type of science, but improving the match between your job, your physical ability, and your capacity to carry out the work. It's about using anatomy, physiology, psychology, and biomechanics to optimize your safety, protect your health, and maximize your comfort—while letting you do your job or go about your everyday life. It sounds complicated, but it's common sense really. Technology and furniture should be designed around your needs—you shouldn't have to fit into what designers decree just because it looks nice. When you sit or lie in positions where the natural curves of your spine are preserved, there is less compression of your intervertebral discs and less strain on your back.

Here's an idea for you...

Avoid computer hump. Fix the height of your screen when working with any PC so that the center is parallel to your eyes. Check that the height of your desk lets your shoulders relax and keeps your elbows at right angles, as elevating your arms to type will really put your intervertebral discs under pressure. Sit up straight, close to your desk, and square toward it. Adjust the height of your chair relative to your desk with your feet flat on the ground.

MATCHMAKING—YOU AND YOUR JOB

If you get the ergonomics right in your workplace you're less likely to get back pain. You and your employers need to think about how you sit, move, and lift at work. You need to have good posture and be able to handle weighty loads correctly so that there's the least amount of strain on your spine. Work surfaces should allow enough clearance for your legs so you can sit or stand comfortably.

DON'T TAKE A CHANCE

You might get away with sitting in a rickety chair or at a poorly designed desk when it's an occasional event. But do it regularly and you'll suffer, baby.

Reaching into a stretched position once in a while is easy and normally not a problem—let's face it, it's what all those joints and hinges on your body are about, right?—but maintaining such a position for even quite a short period can strain your back. Postural strains can cause damage when they occur many times in a day, or over long periods. So, while it may be no problem for someone to bend down to knee height to collect a document emerging from a printer once, printing out *War and Peace* one page at a time is a serious no-no.

SITTING COMFORTABLY?

You'll no doubt be sitting at your computer for hours at a time, so make sure your chair gives good support to your lumbar spine. Most people prefer to sit leaning back in a chair. Unfortunately, most workstations don't let you do this in a supported way. Get a seat with an adjustable backrest. A chair with armrests lets you sit and relax your back and elbows from time to time. It's good to be able to alter the angle of the seat, too. Remember, there's more than one comfortable position.

Sit up straight instead of slouching and putting strain on your back. Your wrists should be straight while you tap lightly on the keyboard. Position the keyboard so that the letter "B" is opposite your belly button and sit square to the desk and computer screen. Keeping your mouse near to your keyboard will prevent unnecessary stretching and enable you to retain a good posture while you use it.

WORKING WITH YOUR LAPTOP

You'll need to take more frequent breaks when working from your laptop—say, every hour or so—since you can't adjust the height of the screen as you can with a desktop computer (apart from lifting it up and down, of course). You could always use a laptop cushion to raise it to the correct height. You know it's the right height if you can see the screen with your neck straight.

If you have to lean over a bench, a forward tilt to your chair seat will allow your pelvis to tilt slightly, too, enabling you to maintain the curve of your lumbar spine. If you can't alter the angle of your seat, add a wedge of foam, as in IDEA 11, *Take a stand or sit tight.*

Try another idea...

"A desk is a dangerous place from which to watch the world."
JOHN LE CARRÉ

Defining idea...

How did it go?

Q **How can I convince my boss that it's worth thinking of the ergonomic aspects of my job?**

A   *A good employer won't want trained workers calling in sick with a bad back. In a packing department, for example, the position of a conveyer belt can be adjusted at minimal expense to prevent too much regular twisting. Are you or others being expected to do too much activity before taking a rest? Look at the equipment you use and the furniture where you sit or work: Does it suit your body size? Can you see and hear all you need to (NOT including office gossip) without moving awkwardly? Does the equipment or system cause you discomfort if you use it for any length of time?*

6

Ooh, you don't want to do that...

Unless you have the physique of Atlas, you'd better learn how to lift weight in a way that protects your back from strain.

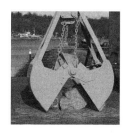

Eastern European weightlifters probably practice by playing catch the fridge, but for most of us picking up a heavy bag of groceries or moving an item of furniture is enough to put your back out.

THINK BEFORE YOU LIFT

The bottom line is that if you're not confident that you can lift an object safely because it's too heavy or awkward, don't lift it. Don't take the risk. There's always an alternative way to move it without straining or injuring your back. And if there isn't, well, some things are just destined to stay put! The alternatives can even be fun—you could insist on being followed by a moose of a man who does your lifting for you. Or you could take to tottering around on stilettos and refusing to lift a finger except to summon the maitre d'. Admittedly this is harder to pull off if you happen to be male.

Learn the maximum weight you should lift in a variety of situations. Lifting from below knee height or above shoulder height if close to the body should be limited to 22 (15) pounds for men (women); if farther away than the length of your forearm, 11 (7.7) pounds; at waist height, close to the body, 55 (37) pounds. Reduce by 10–20 percent if twisting is involved; if lifting is repeated once or twice per minute, reduce by 20 percent; and if repeated 12 times per minute, reduce by 80 percent.

Sometimes it's not a heavy weight that'll do the damage, but what seems like an easy lift that you do without much thought, especially if your muscles are tired.

There are some situations where you're particularly at risk: twisting at the same time as lifting, or when putting shopping bags in the back of your car, when you are reaching forward with a weight in your arms.

At work, it's the incorrect handling of loads that causes many injuries, resulting in pain, time off work, and even permanent disability. Manual handling regulations apply to moving any weights at work, through lifting, lowering, pushing, pulling, carrying, holding, or moving, whether these movements are done by hand or using other bodily force. They cover the nature of the force applied. That is the duration, frequency, magnitude, and posture you adopt, whether it's an animate load, such as moving people or animals, or inanimate, such as shifting crates. If you think the weights you're being asked to lift at work are too heavy or awkward, then ask your union or manager for an assessment under the manual handling regs. That will startle them!

Defining idea...

"Lifting a barbell ain't like eating no watermelon."
TOAD, Olympic weightlifter

It may seem to you that you don't do "lifting" at work anyway. But if your job doesn't normally involve physical effort, you are probably more vulnerable if you're unexpectedly required to lift something such as a box of photocopier paper than someone who handles heavy weights every day.

HOW SHOULD I LIFT, THEN?

Use a straight back/bent knees posture to hold an object close to your body so that it can fit between your knees while you are lifting it. That way, the weight you're lifting exerts less leverage on your spine. Get into the habit of bending your knees rather than your back when you go to lift something, hold the object close in toward your body, and avoid twisting sideways at the same time as you lift.

When you carry a load you compress your intervertebral discs. This is not usually a problem if the natural curves of the spine are maintained. But if your back is bent forward or sideways or twisted, an uneven stress is placed on one part of your discs or the ligaments around them, and damage may occur. Loads carried nearer the spine are easier to control, and create less strain on the spine. Twisting, stooping, or reaching upward with a load places more strain on the spine. Loads that are awkward, bulky, prone to shift, or have to be handled in limited spaces or with poor lighting are particularly hazardous.

Avoid lifting objects that are too heavy. If possible, minimize their weight by splitting them into separate loads. Only lift objects that can be held close to your body. If you can't hold an object close, then use some sort of handling aid. Push rather than pull objects lying on the floor.

Developing strong abdominal muscles will reduce the strain on your lumbar spine, with the muscles effectively splinting the spine from the front. Look at IDEA 8, *Home goals*, for guidance on this.

Try another idea...

Keep your back in shape with regular exercise. IDEA 7, *Keeping active*, gives hints on how swimming will strengthen your back muscles.

...and another

25

How did
it go?

Q **I can't avoid lifting my groceries—my family has the appetite of a pack of professional wrestlers and if I don't keep them fueled they'll probably eat the furniture. What else can I do?**

A   *First up, don't overload your shopping bags. Fully laden, they should be no heavier than 7.5 pounds (women) or 11 pounds (men). Weigh this out at home so you know what it feels and looks like. Next, make sure there's enough room in your car for you to lift loads in and out without twisting. Consider buying a hatchback if you don't have one already. Finally, why not take your voracious family with you to help with the lifting; you can always leave them in the car if you don't trust them to behave themselves in the supermarket.*

Q **Is your "bent knees/straight back" advice sufficient for someone like me who is a couch potato?**

A   *No, it probably isn't—but it's a start! Improving your general fitness will help to strengthen your back and keep it flexible, and will thereby help prevent back problems; but it will require a little effort from you, if you feel up to it.*

7

Keeping active

Addicted to exercise? Craving your regular fix? If not, you should be. Exercise on as many days per week as possible—and avoid withdrawal symptoms altogether with a daily workout.

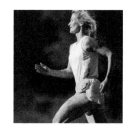

Binge exercising on the weekends is okay, but not as good as regular daily activity. So indulge in multiple rounds of golf or sets of tennis, but walk, bike, or go to the gym in the meantime.

DO I HAVE TO?

Far too many people are fat slobs. Fifty years ago you'd have used as much energy in your job or at home doing the domestic work as if you were running a marathon race every single week. How times have changed! The average person now watches over 26 hours of television a week (that's one for every mile). Children spend many hours watching videos or playing computer games (and adults, too) rather than getting off their butts and running around. We use cars to travel everywhere because we are so short of time. Many jobs involve sitting at a desk, and most of us get no exercise at work other than regular visits to the coffee machine and the morning trek to pick up the doughnuts.

Here's an idea for you...

Increase the amount of activity in your daily routine. Do more gardening, or do it with more gusto—actually digging over the garden as often as the experts suggest. When you go shopping, park your car farther away, or walk to the store instead of driving for small items that you can easily carry. Tackle your housework with more effort— spring clean your rooms more than once a decade, or tidy up the garage and shed and keep them in order in the future. Don't pay someone else to do the decorating or gardening for you—do it yourself for the extra activity and satisfaction you'll get.

On the other hand, we stuff ourselves with food and drink as much as we ever did. So, even though we are getting far less exercise, we are still packing in just as many calories. Result? We're more likely to be overweight or obese these days. And being inactive increases your risk of heart disease and stroke. So do something about it.

KEEP ACTIVE

That's a key message for beating back pain. This means keep doing normal everyday activities if you've got back pain, not sitting around resting. You don't have to be the defensive tackle in a pick-up football game or do a two-hour workout in the gym, but you do have to put more into it than the odd Roger Moore–esque heavy-duty eyebrow lift.

BUILD UP SLOWLY

Increase the amount of exercise you do each day gradually—blitzing it will only lead to injury. Don't go for sports that involve twisting, like hockey and squash, until you have already regained some fitness/suppleness and feel your back can take it.

Work toward doing 30 minutes of moderate intensity activity on at least 5 days of the week. The 30 minutes can be accumulated throughout the day in

10–15 minute bouts. Moderate intensity means breathing slightly harder than normal but still being within your "comfort zone." You should be able to continue the activity while talking at the same time. That will please the gossips amongst you!

Get out there and enjoy the countryside—it's just waiting for you to discover it. Take a look at IDEA 26, *Get a life*, and get with it.

Try another idea...

Extend some of your exercise sessions to 45 minutes or more. This will encourage your body to use some of your fat stores as a source of energy.

CUT DOWN THE AMOUNT OF TIME YOU SPEND SITTING AROUND

Try not to sit down for more than 30 minutes at a time. That might mean cutting down on those 3-hour videos—or pause the video and take a walking break.

USE LARGE MUSCLE GROUPS

The best activities for boosting your weight loss and fitness are those involving large muscle groups. These are mainly aerobic exercises: walking, running, swimming, or cycling. You can read up on how much energy various exercises use, given as the equivalent in calories per hour.

Doing weight-bearing exercises, such as walking and climbing a hill (or mountain— or even the stairs!), helps to build up your muscles. This maintains your strength and is a good way to keep your back muscles well honed. Different types of exercise suit different people, so try various activities to find out what suits your back best.

"Muscles come and go. Flab lasts."
BILL VAUGHAN, journalist

Defining idea...

29

DON'T OVERDO IT

Pace yourself. As a new convert to the benefits of exercise it is tempting to go overboard and be exercising every spare minute of your day. You won't be able to keep it up, you'll get bored, and you'll slink back to the TV or the bar. It's not all or nothing—settle for a halfway position and enjoy the best of both worlds.

How did it go?

Q   Sounds like I'm going to have to grit my teeth and make myself do some regular exercise, even if there's bad weather and I don't feel like it. Where's the fun in that?

A   *You won't continue with regular exercise unless you enjoy doing it—or you're a masochist. So experiment with what kind of exercise fits your lifestyle, and what you like doing. When exercise is a pleasure, fitness is easy. A good spin-off might be the new friends you meet while doing your new physical activity. And the happier you are, the better your back will be.*

Q   I'm so injury-prone that I spend more time in the club bar than on the field. Any tips on making sure I don't end up worse off from doing exercise than I started out?

A   *If you're doing any sports, you need to warm up first. And cool down slowly at the end of a game by doing a few exercises before resting. Don't just slump in a chair afterward. Avoid exercise that jars your spine, like jogging on hard pavement—and avoid the bar afterward!*

8

Home goals

The object of this exercise is to prevent and treat your back problems. That's your goal. You'll have to work at it. But it will be worth it.

Learn exercises to treat yourself and avoid time off work, expensive medicines, or costly therapy. It's amazing what you can do with a wall, a floor, and the know-how.

EXERCISES FOR A SLIPPED DISC

You'll need to concentrate on this one. If your pain is in the center of your lumbar spine (if it is, the pain travels from the center of your back around your waistline area), you should lie on the floor with your hands under your shoulders. Make sure you are facedown first. Then push yourself up until your arms are straight, leaving your hips on the floor. At the ninth or tenth movement, you should try to relax the muscles around your lumbar spine so that your hips sag to the floor. Try lying on your front for 15–20 minutes while you're watching television or reading. Alternatively, if you have neck problems, too, or you can't get down on the floor, you can stand astride (standing upright with your legs straight and feet apart 20 inches or so) and lean backward 10 times with your hands on your waist.

Here's an idea for you... **Join a back school where a physiotherapist teaches exercises. A typical class for a group of people with back problems will include strengthening and stretching exercises, a relaxation session, and some brief education about back care. If you go along to a class for a month or two you'll notice the difference in controlling your back pain for up to a year afterward.**

If your pain spreads down one side of your body—into your butt, thigh, or lower leg—you should try to compress your spine on the painful side. Leaning this way may seem illogical—the natural tendency is to lean away from the painful side or to slouch in a chair, as these postures relieve pressure on your nerve roots—but such relief is only temporary and hinders your recovery by keeping the disc out of position.

Now stand astride beside a wall with the painful side away from it, resting your elbow against the wall. Then glide your hips in toward the wall ten times. So, if your back pain is sited on your left side, lean to the left (and similarly for the right). The pain should lessen, or move upward and toward the center of your back. If this standing exercise doesn't do the trick, there is an alternative. Lie facedown on the floor with your arms in the push-up position. Now make a sideways kink in your spine with your hips shifted away from the painful side and do ten push-ups with first bent and then straightened arms, leaving your hips on the floor. Do ten of these movements every hour for the first two days, to try to move the disc back into a central position.

If neither of these series of movements helps, rotating your spine may be the answer. Lie on your back with your knees bent and roll your knees over toward the painful side. Leave them there for 2–3 minutes before returning them to the center position. Repeat this maneuver 3–4 times. Once the pain has moved from your leg to the middle of your back, do the exercises for central back pain. When the pain has settled, maintain your back in prime condition by doing ten leaning backward movements every day.

Read more about Pilates to help develop your abdominal muscles in IDEA 20, *At the core of the matter.*

Try another idea...

AND THERE'S MORE

The back is not the be-all and end-all of useful exercises—your abdomen also needs attention. Lie on the floor, bend your knees, preferably placing your calves on a stool, then lift up your head to look at your knees. As you become stronger, you may be able to reach forward and eventually sit up. There's a deep corset-like muscle running round your abdomen, the transversus muscle, which you can exercise by tensing your navel toward your spine. You can identify and isolate this muscle when on your hands and knees with your tummy hanging down (assuming it doesn't drag on the ground). As you tense your navel your transversus muscle moves up toward your spine—feel it with one hand. Don't do sit-ups by fixing your feet under a piece of furniture with your legs out straight in front of you. That'll put too much strain on the discs of your spine.

There are also diagonal muscles to exercise, and reaching down to the outside of each of your thighs will work those. You can tone up the muscles at the side of your abdomen by lying on your side and lifting your upper leg. You should start with ten of each movement a few times a day, gradually increasing the number every few days as you become stronger.

"Every man is the architect of his own fortune."
SALLUST

Defining idea...

How did
it go?

Q How can I strengthen my muscles to keep back pain away?

A   *As you recover from your back pain episode, continue with your exercises, stretching backward. Strengthen the muscles that do this movement by lying on your front and lifting your head, hands, and shoulders off the ground. The exercise can be made more difficult as you become stronger by putting your hands under your forehead.*

Q When I did exercises for my back muscles, the pain got worse instead of better. Am I malformed, or did I do something wrong?

A   *Not necessarily (to both questions!). Sometimes, as the bout of exercise pushes the jelly back into the center of the disc, the extra volume creates a temporary shot of pain. This will settle, so long as the pain is moving up toward the center of your spine. If the pain moves down instead, stop doing the exercises that cause the pain and consult a physiotherapist or doctor to be reassessed.*

9

Full scream ahead

It can be a real pain to do the chores. But it needn't be. Do your homework and you'll find ways to remove the strain.

Just because you've got a back problem doesn't mean you can get out of doing the chores. Maybe you can afford a cleaner, but maybe it's you who does it all...

Whatever your circumstances, there'll always be some jobs that crop up at home or in the garden that are up to you. Even if you've got a daily cleaner, a visiting friend might spill a drink on the carpet, or you may have to wash and iron a fancy outfit for an unexpected night out (lucky you!).

IRONING

Ensure that the ironing board is adjusted to the correct height. If it won't go high enough, buy one that will—they're not expensive and the comfort factor is well worth it. Try keeping your weight spread evenly on both your feet. Using a steam setting means that you can apply a lighter pressure to the clothes as you iron them. Several short sessions of ironing are better than one lengthy one (so long as you remember to go back!). Oh yes, and perching on a stool may help your back, too.

Here's an idea for you... **Clean up your act. Use a ladder when you're cleaning windows and don't balance on boxes or other precarious objects. Move the steps or ladder rather than stretch out too far and put strain on your back. Only half fill a bucket with water, so that it's not so heavy to carry. Several short sessions of cleaning windows are better than pushing yourself to do the entire job at once.**

VACUUM CLEANING

Using an upright vacuum cleaner means less bending down than with a cylinder type. On the minus side, a standard upright may be heavier to push around, though there are lightweight varieties. Get help moving large pieces of furniture, such as beds, so you can vacuum underneath them and avoid twisting your body—why should you struggle alone? Your back's too precious.

An upright cleaner with a long hose can reach up to twelve stairs at a time rather than the seven stairs for most upright cleaners. This'll save you from having to balance the vacuum cleaner on the stairs with one hand while twisting to clean the next few stairs with the other.

DUSTING/MAKING BEDS/CLEANING TUBS

Kneel down for these sorts of chores. That way, you'll create less strain on your spine than when stooping over and bending your back. Bend your knees or kneel to tuck in sheets. To clean the tub, bend your hips and knees and keep your back straight. Don't flip heavy duvets over the bed; take your time to roll them over.

WATCHING TV/READING/SEWING/KNITTING

It's best to sit directly in front of the TV rather than twisting to view the screen. Sit up straight in a chair with good support rather than slumping into a soft, "comfy" chair. Don't let your head droop when you're knitting, sewing, or reading as your spine will be hunched. Get up and move around frequently—though not to go and eat snacks.

SHOPPING

Use a cart rather than a basket, so you're not carrying a load unnecessarily. But avoid those broken ones with stiff wheels that can jolt or twist your spine as you try to maneuver them around the store. Don't load so much into your cart that pushing it is a Herculean task. Be careful when you're lifting the goods out of your basket or cart at the checkout, or transferring them into your car or unloading them at home. When carrying, even out your load by using two bags and holding one in each hand.

STORAGE

Don't store heavy objects on the floor. They may be safe, but it's a real strain picking them up from floor level instead of waist height.

DO-IT-YOURSELF JOBS

Pick tools that are right for the job so you don't trigger your back pain. Small jobs at a bench at waist height will mean no awkward bends to the ground. Use electrically activated tools rather than your brawn whenever possible. Don't stick at one job for too long—swap between activities so that you're not straining your back or one particular joint unduly.

Pace yourself to your own level of fitness in the garden. Spread out the gardening over days or weeks. Do some gentle exercises or stretching before you start so that your body's ready for it. Check out IDEA 41, *Everything's coming up roses,* **for some really earthy ideas on gardening.**

Try another idea...

"Housework's the hardest work in the world. That's why men won't do it."
EDNA FERBER, novelist

Defining idea...

37

How did it go?

Q   Christmas is great. But the Christmas chores are even greater! Any tips?

A   *Pace yourself and prepare well in advance. Rest every so often when doing a long job. Better still, change tasks and do something else that uses a different set of muscles. Plan how overnight guests will sleep so that you don't end up on a makeshift bed that triggers your back pain. Having an oven at waist height will mean you don't have to lift the turkey from down near the floor to table height. If you haven't got one, put it on your Christmas list. Don't lift heavy pans from the back burners of your stovetop— keep them at the front.*

Q   I get a backache stooping over when doing the dishes because we have such a low sink. We can't afford to replace the sink, and my partner won't let me get away with just supervising—so what else can I do?

A   *Why not raise your kitchen sink by placing an upturned bowl beneath it? You can also open the cabinet under the sink and place one foot on the bottom shelf, or put your foot on a stool. That'll keep your back straight while you lean over.*

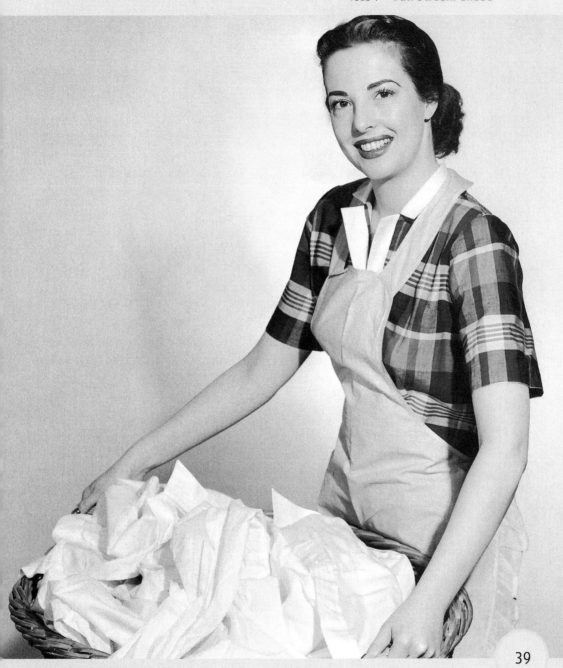

39

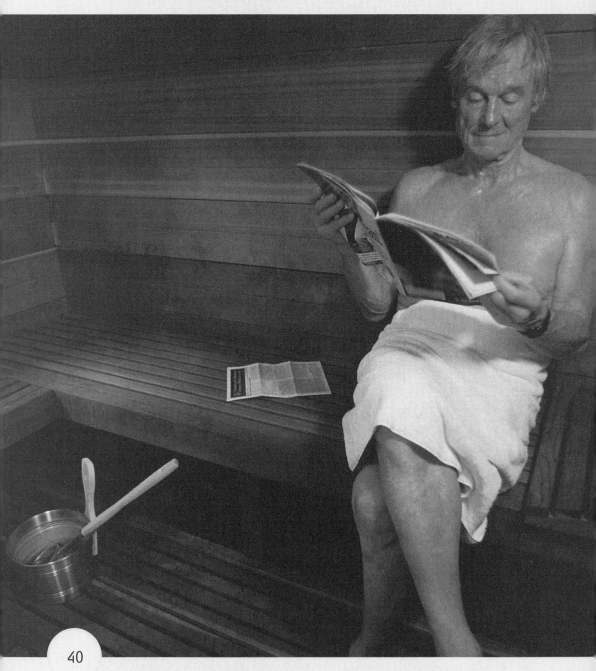

10

Some like it hot

What do frozen peas, a wheat bag, and a sauna have in common? They can all help to relieve your back pain.

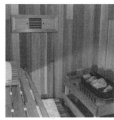

Do you go hot and cold just thinking about how much your back hurts sometimes? Well, why not try out heat or ice to find out how much they could help?

ICE BREAKER

An ice pack can be made by wrapping crushed ice or a bag of frozen peas (or beans; it's your choice) in a thin cloth such as a tea towel. Hold it against the painful area of your back (or any other part that hurts) for 5–10 minutes only. If doing this relieves your symptoms, then repeat the treatment 3 times a day. Remember to put the frozen peas back into the freezer between times. Don't eat the peas at a later date, as they'll have been defrosted and refrozen many times and your guts may suffer. If they do, get an ice pack…

Instead of messing around with melting ice cubes, why not buy a fluid-filled pack that cools itself down by chemical reaction? Squeezing and massaging the outside of the pack kick-starts the reaction. Or you can buy bags of gel that you store in the freezer so that they're always cold and ready for use. Avoid ice burn by rubbing baby oil on your bare skin or wearing light clothing before applying the pack.

How it works is that the ice pack causes the blood vessels near the surface of your skin to constrict, to stop your body from losing heat. The blood then circulates more deeply in your tissues. However, to prevent that area of your body from getting frostbite, after 5–10 minutes the blood vessels near the skin open up again. This draws the blood from deep down to the surface of your skin, with fresh blood from elsewhere in your body replacing that from your deeper tissues, boosting nutrition and healing in that area of your body. If you have any muscles in spasm, the cold also helps them to relax. If you don't believe that something so simple as an ice pack can work so well, give it a try next time you're in pain.

HEAT

Heat works by getting your blood vessels to open up as warmth seeps through. This increases blood flow in the area, improving nutrition and the healing effects from a good blood supply. Gentle warmth also helps to relieve muscle spasm as the muscles relax. Heat or warmth also seems to soothe your nerve endings so that they're less susceptible to irritation from movement or pressure.

"Every road has two directions."
RUSSIAN PROVERB

A hot water bottle wrapped in a towel is cheap, easy, and effective. Alternatively, there are a variety of heat-giving packs that you can buy or make. A wheat bag or gel-containing pack can be heated up in a microwave to the desired temperature and then popped on your painful area immediately. These are available from most pharmacies, health shops, and some supermarkets. You can also get electric heating pads, and some handheld massagers have an infrared warming device incorporated in them. But take care not to burn yourself while handling the heat source or leaving it against your back.

Escape to IDEA 40, *A day in your life*, to find out how great saunas are as another source of warmth.

Try another idea...

Infrared lamps are useful for heat treatment—but they are expensive and no more effective than the cheaper methods. Don't use ultraviolet or sunlamps, as you'll just get sunburn to go with your backache. Having said that, some sunlamps do have an infrared as well as an ultraviolet facility, so if you do use one, make sure it's on the right setting!

GO FOR WARMTH

Wrap up warm. It may seem like an old wives' tale that a cold wind will give you aches and pains, but back pain does get worse in cold weather as the surrounding muscles tighten up. Put an extra sweater on, and make sure that you don't have a gap between your shirt or sweater and the top of your skirt or pants. Leave the bare midriff for midsummer.

"He that is warm thinks all so."
ENGLISH PROVERB

Defining idea...

43

Why not try a hot bath? Oooh, lovely! Soaking in a hot bath when you've got back pain—marvelous! But make sure you're not slumping in the tub. So really, a hot shower might be better. Another answer is to use the Jacuzzi or hydrotherapy pool at a gym or health spa to get heat on your back. Some of them have chairs heated by warm water dribbling down that might suit you well. Steam baths are worth trying, too. Visit your local health spa or gym and try out their steam room.

How did it go?

Q   Is it a case of the hotter the better to relieve my back pain?

A   *The temperature of your heat pack should create a comfortable warm feeling. If that doesn't relieve the pain, then making it hotter and hotter won't be any more likely to work—and you might blister or burn yourself, creating new troubles. My rule of thumb is "If you smell cooking, stop."*

Q   Do the smelly rubs work? I don't want to use them if they could be harmful.

A   *They seem to work in the same way that heat packs work—by opening up the blood vessels under your skin. This increases the blood supply and thereby brings more nutrition to the area, thus helping the healing process. I think the fact that you'll smell like a wrestler's jockstrap is just an added bonus.*

Take a stand or sit tight

Look to your feet and survey your seat. A lumbar support may be just the sort of crutch you need for your pain to recede.

Go catalog shopping for things to help you sit or stand more comfortably. You don't have to do everything yourself—there are some great gadgets and aids to help you.

FEET FIRST

Shoe insoles help some people with mild back pain. The position of your feet affects the curvature of your spine. If you've got flat feet the hollow of the curve of your lower spine is increased—and this strains your ligaments. Shaped insoles can correct your flat-footed posture and thus relieve your backache. The first step is to get a proper podiatric assessment if your feet are painful. Your podiatrist can then provide you with shaped insoles for your specific problem. Otherwise, buy a set of off-the-shelf insoles from a pharmacy.

Here's an idea for you... **If your chair doesn't tilt forward, sit on a triangular wedge of foam. Whether you buy one or make your own, it should be about 10 inches square with a 2-inch drop from back to front. Sitting on this will tilt your pelvis forward and help maintain your lumbar curve. It's even more important in cars, as often your knees are higher than your bottom, which pushes your back into a curved position.**

If high heels are your thing, don't forget that they can strain your spine because they alter your center of gravity and the whole mechanics of your lower back. And if you're tottering about, you might be unstable and twist the muscles of your back in an effort to remain upright. So keep your high heels for occasional use and short distances. And make sure you've got a ride home so you won't have to walk.

Don't struggle if you don't have to. Slip-on shoes are easier for you to wear if you've got back pain since you don't have to fasten any laces.

STICK TO IT

Walking sticks, elbow crutches, and walking frames all help to spread your body load between your legs and arms and reduce the pressure on the nerves in your spine. So using one of these should decrease your pain. A stick keeps you upright and counteracts any muscle imbalance if your pain means you have an abnormal posture from muscle spasms. You can buy a walking stick from a pharmacy; for the others you'll need a catalog or specialist shop. Or your physiotherapist could supply what you need from her clinic.

LUMBAR BRACE

A lumbar brace can boost the strength of your abdominal muscles and limit the movement of your lower back. Of course, it's just for short-term use. If you wear a lumbar brace for too long, you'll be stuck with it—by not using your own muscles, they'll waste away. (It's a shame they haven't developed a beer-belly brace...)

Some cars have an adjustable lumbar support incorporated into the car seat. Turning the handle exaggerates the curve of the seat to fit your lower back shape. See IDEA 5, *Ergonomics—pure science*, for more hints on ergonomics and comfortable seating.

Try another idea...

LUMBAR SUPPORT

Lumbar supports for your spine help to keep it in a good position, keeping the curve at the correct angle when you're sitting or driving a car. A lumbar roll is a sausage-shaped cushion, typically of covered foam. An adjustable elastic strap means you can fix it to your chair at the right level. You should be able to get one from your local pharmacy, a catalog, or maybe even a car accessory shop.

MOLDED SEAT

A portable seat insert that's designed to provide a well-positioned back curve to support your spine is also available. It's a two-piece molded seat with adjustable hinges. You sit on one part and the second part lies against your back. Place it on any seat that has a back to it for instant support.

" 'Tis not enough to help the feeble up but to support him after."
WILLIAM SHAKESPEARE

Defining idea...

GADGETS FOR DAILY LIVING

Try using a "helping hand" gadget to pick up objects lying on the floor. It's like a litter picker. You can buy one from general stores, pharmacies, or shops selling disability equipment. Use a long shoehorn so you don't have to bend down to pull your shoes on. Another gadget can help you put on your socks, stockings, or tights for when you're in extreme pain and want to avoid moving any more than necessary. A bath seat will mean not having to lower your bottom down so far (though you might not be able to pull the plug out so easily).

AIDS TO EXERCISE

There's lots of equipment out there designed to exercise particular parts of your body. For instance, an ab roller is a frame that supports your neck as you work your abdominal muscles and is particularly useful for people with lower back pain.

Q **I'm a first-time jogger. Should I wear insoles in my shoes?**

How did it go?

A *If you're playing sports or running marathons, you should buy shock-absorbing insoles to reduce the jarring on your spine. There's a greater jarring effect when you run on roads than when you run on grass, commonly attributed to the harder surface. Modern treadmills are usually sprung to prevent the jarring, so they may be a safer option for jogging rather than thumping the pavement or country lanes.*

Q **My friend loaned me his lumbar brace, which is not how I'd imagined it. Are there different types?**

A *There's a variety. Most are worn next to your skin or on top of your underwear, though some go over work clothes to support you when doing heavy work. Then there's the weightlifter's belt, a Neoprene sports support, or a specially made brace with metal struts. They are usually readily available through catalogs, sports shops, and shops specializing in disability aids and equipment, or through an occupational health supplier in your place of work. You can also buy a back support belt from a pharmacy to give your back and abdominal muscles some limited support and warmth, but remember to use it only in the short term.*

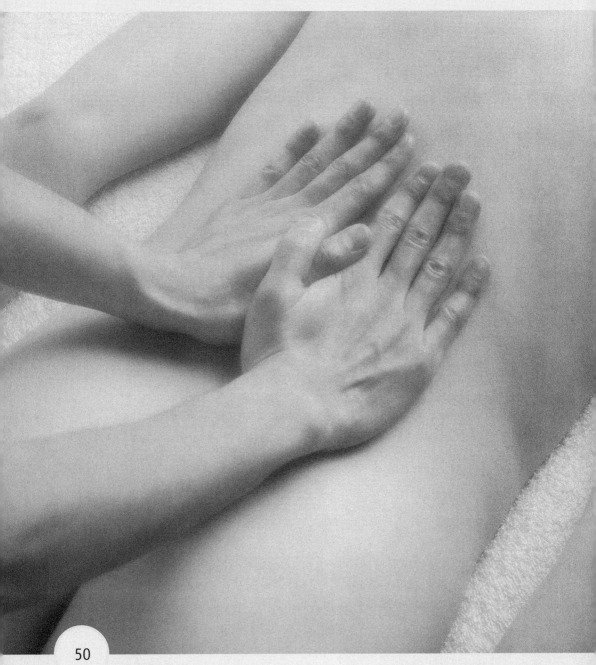

12

What's the alternative?

We're all fazed by the alternatives: What ad to believe or which recommendation to go for. Do you opt for a doctor's advice or the therapist's kindly hands or some tasty potions?

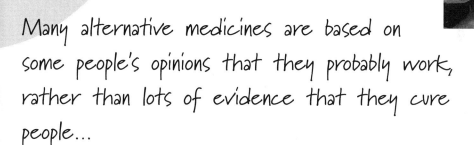

Many alternative medicines are based on some people's opinions that they probably work, rather than lots of evidence that they cure people...

WHO PROVIDES ALTERNATIVE MEDICINE?

Some alternative medicine practitioners are practicing health professionals, such as doctors, physiotherapists, or nurses who are state registered with their own professional bodies. Others, such as osteopaths and chiropractors, are registered with their own statutory bodies.

Most alternative medicine practitioners have completed further education in their discipline. Their knowledge and skills mainly come from training based on what's been passed down by tradition rather than proven by scientific evidence.

Here's an idea for you... Go ahead—opt for a hands-on treatment. Many of the alternatives involve other people touching you with their hands. The exclusive attention of a therapist will make you feel good and cared for, if not loved. You'll leave an alternative therapy session immediately feeling marvelous, as opposed to conventional health care, when you might leave with a prescription for a drug that promises benefits for the future.

HOW DOES IT WORK?

There are some common features between the various kinds of alternative therapies. Many holistic practitioners view human illness as resulting from a combination of physical, psychological, social, and spiritual problems. They believe in the body's capacity for self-repair. Each person is treated as an individual. Their package of care therefore includes advice about lifestyle, counseling, relaxation, diet, and exercise, as well as the therapy for troublesome symptoms.

Some of the terms used by holistic practitioners, such as *oi/chi* or *prana* energy, have no equivalent in Western medical culture. Such energy travels through channels—*chakras* or meridians—as in acupuncture.

Diseases of specific organs or systems of the body can be linked to particular mental or emotional patterns of symptoms. Anxiety and fear might cause digestive disturbances—as you'll know from the morning of an exam or important interview. Holistic treatments try to clear and balance these disturbed energies by working on the body's self-healing capacity to provoke a positive immune response rather than targeting specific symptoms or diseases.

Many conventional health professionals practice in this holistic manner, too. The holistic approach sees everyone as unique. Scientific, artistic, and spiritual insights need to be applied together to restore health. The loss of a sense of meaning and purpose in your life may lead to a deterioration in your health—so that alternative medicines generally involve psychosocial aspects, too. Holistic practitioners believe that illness provides opportunities for positive change as you reflect on your circumstances and create a better balance to your life. There are lots of reasons why people try alternative medicine, but one is that some are low tech.

Interested in being rubbed up the right way? See IDEA 13, *Hands on,* **to find out what it entails.**

Try another idea...

Why not extract the goodness from IDEA 22, *Find your roots,* **and concoct your own pain-busting remedy?**

...and another

THE FEEL-GOOD FACTOR

Some people try alternative medicines because they're desperate. If you're stuck with back pain after trying everything that your doctors have suggested, you'll probably be willing to give anything a try. You may be skeptical about the benefits or dangers of conventional treatments prescribed by doctors. The feeling of being in control of the various treatments because you're paying appeals to some people. There are so many different approaches that, as long as you can afford it, you should find something to help you.

Defining
idea...

"Above all, remember that the most important thing you can take anywhere is not a Gucci bag or French-cut jeans; it's an open mind."
GAIL RUBIN BERNY

DOES IT WORK?

We don't know how many of the alternative therapies are effective for which conditions. Just because acupuncture is effective for lower back pain doesn't necessarily mean that it's effective for headaches. For many people it's the placebo effect, the fact that they're taking a treatment, that makes them think the treatment is working. If someone listens to you with interest and uses their hands to massage or treat you, you're likely to leave that consultation feeling better. But if it works, don't knock it.

MIX 'N' MATCH

If you're skeptical of the alternatives or unwilling to forgo conventional medicine, you could try herbal medicines and conventional health care with the same practitioner. See if they've got a prospectus explaining what's offered. For example, you could take painkillers as well as trying osteopathy. Don't go to more than one practitioner at a time, though—their treatments might conflict.

Q   **I'm confused. There are so many alternative medicines to choose from when you look at the ads. How many are there?**

How did it go?

A   *There are more than one hundred forms of alternative medicine for back pain. Some of the most popular are acupuncture, manipulation, massage and aromatherapy, chiropractic, osteopathy, reflexology, herbal medicine, and homeopathy. Some are an alternative to conventional health care, while others, like aromatherapy, homeopathy, and acupuncture, may be available from your usual health care service as an integral part of your treatment.*

Q   **Some alternative medicines sound safer than conventional medicines. Are they?**

A   *Little research has been carried out on these types of therapies. So there's little evidence that they work and little evidence that they don't work, either. Likewise, we don't know enough about how safe the various alternative medicines are. We need more reliable information before we can say for sure which are safe and effective. On the other hand, conventional medicines have been tried and tested—and their shortfalls and side effects noted. Whether you stick with the devil you know is up to you.*

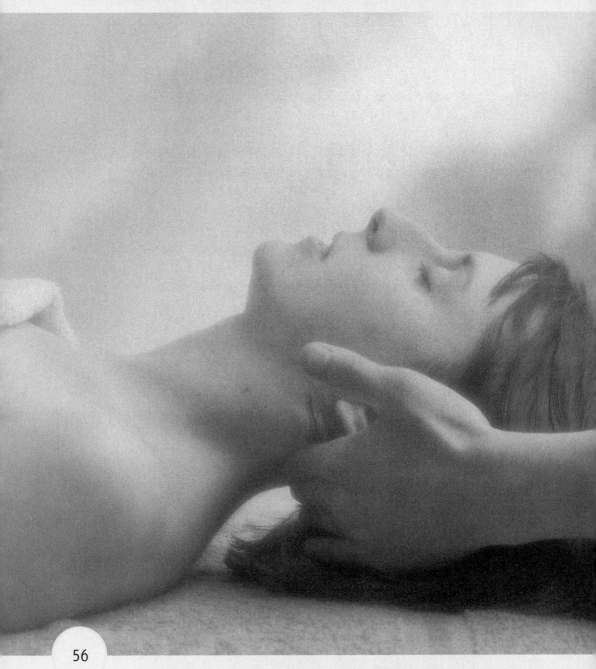

13

Hands on

If you think that massage is all about being caressed and soothed, then try Swedish, Shiatsu, friction, trigger point, Reiki, and Rolfing techniques: They can bring tears to your eyes.

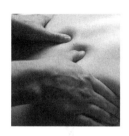

Some of the benefits of massage are from the touch of another person. It's great to feel cared for.

SLIP, SLOP, SLAP

A massage therapist manipulates your body's soft tissues using their hands or a mechanical device to boost your circulation and induce relaxation. This brings about general improvements to your health and relieves muscle spasm or tension in your back, too. Massage induces greater mental and physical relaxation over your whole body—reducing anxiety and boosting well-being. Massage therapists also treat depression and constipation. Most massage sessions last between 15 and 90 minutes.

Here's an idea for you... **Massage begins at home. Buy a back massager with rotating balls that you roll up and down your back with a long, scrubbing brush action—or better still, ask your partner to do it for you. Sit or lie down, close your eyes, and focus on the sensations. That's grrrrrreat.**

HOW DOES MASSAGE WORK?

Mmmm. The stroking, rubbing, kneading, and tapping activities of massage increase your circulation, improve your muscle tone, and relax your body and mind. The improved blood flow increases nutrition and healing to the area being massaged. Massage has other therapeutic effects, too: as a cleanser, by stimulating your lymph circulation, and accelerating the elimination of wastes and toxins.

SWEDISH MASSAGE

The therapist usually massages all of your body, concentrating on one section at a time. They generally work you over systematically, maybe starting on the back and working down to the legs, then, when you turn over, treating your chest, abdomen, shoulders, arms, and face. This is the type of massage usually done in sports centers and health clubs. Emphasis is on the psychological and spiritual aspects of massage.

SPORTS MASSAGE

Sports therapists and others may use massage before and after sporting events. They treat injuries arising from sports activities or other existing problems by using deep massage, coupled with passive and active stretching of various muscle groups.

SHIATSU

This type of therapy dates back to 500 BC. It's a type of massage that concentrates on particular points rather than the whole body, to rebalance the flow of *chi* that circulates around the body. The palms and thumbs are used to apply pressure to the skin at places that often correspond to acupoints—and it may well act like acupuncture, stimulating certain meridians and the body to help itself. Normally clients lie on a futon or table for the treatment. Wear loose clothing, like sweatpants and a T-shirt. No oil is used.

REIKI

Reiki is a kind of touch therapy. The practitioner places his hands on parts of your body near the site of the problem, such as your back. This encourages healing energy to flow through his hands. Sessions last for about an hour, during which time you'll experience deep relaxation and reach a meditative state—which is great for your mental health. But it shouldn't be performed on anyone who's suffering from a serious psychosis, except with the permission of their psychiatrist.

Many massage practitioners use oils as part of the treatment simply to help their hands move over your body. But your practitioner could use the essential oils of aromatherapy as an integral part of the massage. See IDEA 15, *Ahead by a nose*, for more aromatherapeutic suggestions.

Try another idea...

59

ROLFING

This deep massage technique will rebalance your body by bringing your head, shoulders, chest, pelvis, and legs into proper vertical alignment so that you feel more supple. To carry out this deep massage, the therapist applies pressure with his fingers, hands, knuckles, or elbows to lengthen and release the connective tissues of different sites of your body. A bad back should be improved at the same time. Therapy usually consists of at least ten sessions focused on different parts of your body. It can be painful.

WHO DOES MASSAGE?

Some physiotherapists give massages, but on the whole they leave it to sports masseurs, physical therapists, and other massage practitioners.

There are many organizations that massage practitioners can belong to. The National Certification Board for Therapeutic Massage and Bodywork (www.ncbtmb.com) sets standards of practice within the United States.

WHAT HAPPENS WHEN YOU SEE A MASSAGE PRACTITIONER?

He'll ask about your diet and lifestyle, and any aches and pains you've got. You'll usually lie facedown on a table for a back massage—remaining in your underwear, covered by a sheet. A well-designed massage table will have a hole for your face, to stop your nose from getting squashed and to avoid drooling. The professional massage is strictly asexual—the therapist will steer clear of your genitals.

Q It's my first try at massage. Which oil is best?

A It depends what you want to achieve, really. Ayurvedic oil is thought to have anti-inflammatory properties. Hot medicated oils such as this are massaged into your back muscles. Aromatic oils can be used for their relaxing properties.

Q I'm a little clumsy doing massage on myself: I have friction burns and cramps in equal measure. What technique should I be trying?

A Use your thumb and fingers to look for sore spots along your spine—or other muscle groups elsewhere on your body. Apply reasonable pressure and do a gentle rotating movement.

Q We don't have much spare cash. Are massage pads and massage beds worth buying?

A A recliner chair with a massage setting incorporated into it will feel fantastic when you arrive home from work and your muscles are tense and knotted. Or try rectangular pads to cover your whole back. Or handheld massagers for painful areas may be just the remedy you need and can afford.

How did it go?

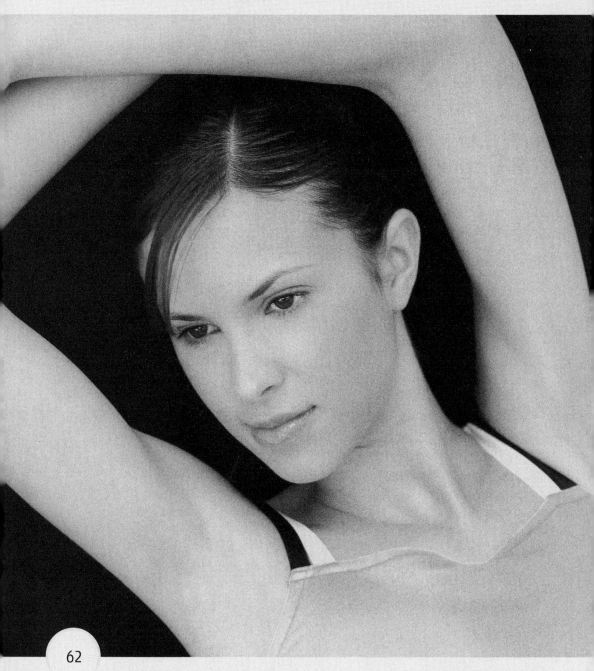

14

Strike a pose

There are plenty of posers strutting their stuff and loving themselves. But not yoga posers. They improve the flow of *prana* energy around their body to obtain harmony of mind, body, and spirit.

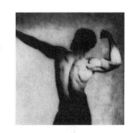

Whether it's upward-facing dog and cat stretches or other positions you favor, yoga can help you to beat your back pain and bring out the animal in you.

YOGA—AN ANCIENT INDIAN SCIENCE

There are several different kinds of yoga, but they all focus on breathing and tranquility. The rationale is that the body and mind cannot function fully if air is not exchanged in the lungs in a proper way. Some yoga movements are gentle while others are physically demanding. Doing yoga sounds lazy, but it really stretches your muscles. Some concentrate on physical postures, while others focus on you controlling your breathing and meditation. Yoga is popular—many celebrities practice yoga and promote its benefits (admittedly, often for money).

At the end of a yoga session, you'll find that the stresses of the day have disappeared, freeing your mind of your daily hassles.

Here's an idea for you...

Try using yoga to strengthen your back muscles. Lie on your front with your palms flat on the floor by your shoulders. Then breathe in and lift up your upper body to look up at the ceiling or sky. Your spine needs to arch back to maintain this posture for 5 seconds with your outstretched arms giving you some support. For a less strenuous version, keep your elbows on the floor and raise your head, rather than the whole of your upper body.

MENTAL AND PHYSICAL BENEFITS

Practicing yoga involves postures, breathing exercises, and meditation aimed at improving your physical and mental functioning. It strengthens your body, improves your general physical fitness, and calms your mind. And you'll certainly notice the effect on your stomach muscles.

Yoga helps to tone up the muscles you use to maintain a good posture. It exercises, rotates, and twists your joints and vertebrae naturally. Hatha yoga is designed to bring the right and left or hot and cold sides of the body into balance. When you're doing a routine workout, the sequence of positions you adopt will provide symmetrical, balanced exercise for your back. The postures you hold are demanding on your muscles. As you focus on particular muscle groups they generate heat, which in turn makes your muscles more flexible. Most of the postures require you to concentrate on the physical positioning of your body, being aware of its axis and balance while clearing your mind of negative thoughts and worries.

Yoga can be used in a preventive way. The various postures contract and tone up many different muscle groups of your body. Quite a few of the postures keep your back flexible and prevent backache. Grabbing and holding the soles of your feet will be followed by complementary bends in another direction, always providing balance.

One way to tackle different muscle groups and stretch your spine is the pelvic tilt. To do this, you lie on your back with your arms by your sides and bend both your knees up so that your ankles are directly below your knees. Keep your feet apart in line with the distance between your hips. Take a deep breath in and raise your pelvis as high as you can, tightening the muscles in your butt and tucking your chin in to touch your chest. Hold that position for five seconds, or less if you find it uncomfortable. Then breathe out and ease your back down onto the floor. Repeat the exercise five times.

There are many other postures and exercises you can do to help your back. Let IDEA 8, *Home goals*, and IDEA 20, *At the core of the matter*, take you through some of these.

Try another idea...

THE SPINE IS THE CENTRAL AXIS OF YOUR BODY

The best position for yoga is when the spine is kept erect. Yoga exercises work on the spine from different angles. The slow-twitching muscles maintain your body's posture. They don't have speed or power, but they do have endurance. This enables them to go about their work slowly without becoming fatigued. The fast-twitching muscles can contract quickly and are reasonably strong, but they fatigue more easily. They are important for fast movements, like running, throwing, typing...

"The art of resting the mind and the power of dismissing from it all care and worry is probably one of the secrets of energy in our great men."
CAPTAIN J. A. HADFIELD

Defining idea...

BEING AWARE OF YOUR BODY

Yoga helps you develop a mental awareness of your body. So, following your yoga exercises, you should maintain that heightened awareness and be less likely to damage yourself as you go about your everyday activities. You'll be more aware of how you're sitting, so you can give yourself a mental slap whenever you slouch.

How did it go?

Q **What's the best way to start yoga—should I just read up on it in a book and get going, or should I find a local class to join?**

A *There are yoga classes for a wide variety of health conditions. If you can find one for arthritis or back pain, you may get more out of it than joining a more general one. Alternatively, you could consult a yoga therapy practitioner for a one-on-one session. It's best not to try yoga after simply reading up on it. If you try a yoga posture using an incorrect position, you could put too much strain on your joints or ligaments. Then you could end up injuring yourself or making your back worse.*

Q **I was gripped by terrible back pain last week. When it happens again can I use yoga to help relax my muscle spasm?**

A *If you're suffering or recovering from a bout of back pain—especially if it's severe—it's best not to take up any form of yoga. Wait until you're better and then go for it.*

66

15

Ahead by a nose

Smell success? That must be the aromatherapy oils overcoming your muscle tension and back pain. You "nose" it'll work for you.

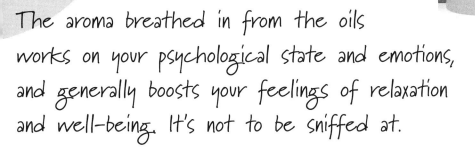

The aroma breathed in from the oils works on your psychological state and emotions, and generally boosts your feelings of relaxation and well-being. It's not to be sniffed at.

TRY IT AND SEE

Try aromatherapy if you want to benefit from the natural healing properties of essential oils. These oils can be extracted from flowers, leaves, fruit, stems, wood, bark, resin, or roots. Essential oils are around 70 times more concentrated than the raw parts of the parent plants. Most are then diluted with vegetable-based oils, though some, such as lavender oil and tea tree oil, can be applied directly on the skin in their pure form. The characteristic aroma and flavor of every plant is due to its essential oils.

Aromatherapy oils are usually massaged into your body. But they can also be added as a few drops to your bath, or used as a perfume, an inhalant, a compress, a vaporizer, or a room spray.

Here's an idea for you...

Use aromatherapy at home by putting oils in your bath or in an oil burner. Or try them in a cold compress held next to your skin. If you massage oil into your back, go over the muscles along the length of your spine (you may need help with this), not just over the painful area. Marjoram, thyme, and ginger are some of the oils used to relieve muscular discomfort and fatigue. Jasmine and sandalwood are relaxing and may help, too.

Aromatherapy is used for pain relief, so try it for your back pain. It's also good for relieving anxiety, nausea, and stress-related conditions. It's generally given as a course of treatment so that the benefits can take root and grow. As time goes by, you'll feel more relaxed, and your back pain will gradually resolve, or at least be kept at bay.

HOW AROMATHERAPY IS CARRIED OUT

"Aesthetic" aromatherapy is carried out as a general treatment at beauty clinics and health spas to create a feeling of well-being. "Holistic" aromatherapy is carried out by trained professionals to treat specific disorders. Some nurses have learned aromatherapy and use this alongside other health treatments in regular clinics or specialized units, such as those providing palliative care to people with terminal illnesses. A holistic approach in aromatherapy is about treating the "whole" person rather than focusing on specific symptoms or health problems.

Typically, you'll lie down on a couch. The aromatherapist will then apply a blend of aromatherapy oils to your body with a full-body massage. Having a massage is probably the best way to have aromatherapy if you're suffering from back pain.

HOW DOES AROMATHERAPY WORK?

Many powers have been attributed to fragrant plants over the centuries. Practitioners believe that the life force of the plant is within the aromatherapy oil, which is then absorbed through the skin or inhaled. Aromatic oils then promote healing and restore the balance between your body and mind. Massage with aromatherapy oils relieves tension in your body and improves your circulation. The effects are exerted as the oil is absorbed through your skin and into your bloodstream to be carried around your body and into your nervous system.

Ask your partner to massage aromatherapy oils into your back regularly. It might become part of your sexual foreplay— see IDEA 31, *"Not tonight, darling—I have a backache,"* for further ideas.

Try another idea...

IS IT DANGEROUS?

Some aromatherapy oils are poisonous if drunk instead of rubbed in or inhaled. So be careful not to leave the bottle where a young child could find it (even if it's not poisonous, it'll be expensive!). The oils should not be applied to damaged skin, so if you're sunburned or have a flare-up of eczema, don't apply it to those areas affected. In fact, you should avoid sunbathing after applying aromatherapy oils to your skin, as you might end up with a dappled effect. It may look good on dalmatians, but then so does fur.

FIND AN AROMATHERAPIST YOU CAN TRUST

Some aromatherapists belong to a professional association, but there's no legal obligation to, and so some don't. It's difficult to be sure how well trained any aromatherapist is—courses can range from a few days to a full university

"There is no need to go to India or anywhere else to find peace. You will find that deep place of silence right in your room, your garden, or even your bathtub."
ELIZABETH KÜBLER-ROSS, psychologist

Defining idea...

69

degree. If they do declare their qualification, go for the BA in therapeutic massage rather than the Dip. in oil.

How did
it go? **Q   I can't afford to visit an aromatherapist, so how do I go about treating myself?**

A   *Add up to seven drops of essential oils to your bath after running the water. Gently agitate the water to disperse the oil evenly. It'll be really relaxing, promise. Or add four to six drops of essential oils into a basin of water to make up a compress. Dip a piece of cloth into the water, squeeze gently, and place over the painful area of your back. Use a hot compress to ease a muscle spasm or a cold one to reduce pain and swelling. Alternatively, you can inhale the oils by adding six to twelve drops of essential oils to a basin of very hot water, then lean over it (carefully, with a straight back) and cover your head with a towel.*

Q   I have diabetes. Is it okay to use aromatherapy oils?

A   *Certain oils suit people with high blood pressure problems, diabetes, epilepsy, or skin irritation better than others. As you suffer from one of these conditions, you should discuss your condition with the aromatherapist so that they can tailor treatment just for you—but don't worry, they will be able to help.*

16

Hang in there

Watch your back—not everyone is your friend. But the therapist who tries traction on your back and relieves your back pain will soon be your best friend.

Although they call it the rack, traction is actually reasonably comfortable. Especially if you do it to somebody else. (Only joking!)

There are no scientific guarantees that traction is effective for lower back pain or for relieving pressure on the nerve roots of your spine. We don't know exactly how much traction force therapists should apply or for how long to treat the various back problems for which it's used. But traction is commonly used by therapists to relieve symptoms of neck and back pain, so someone thinks it must work.

ON THE RACK

Traction is set up on your lumbar spine by passing a strap across your chest and placing a second strap around your pelvis. The strap around your chest is fixed. A weight is then applied to the strap around your pelvis to pull your spine to its full length. This relieves the pressure on the intervertebral discs of your lumbar spine.

Here's an idea for you... **Engage a friend in a little leg pulling. Lie on your back on the floor. Ask your friend to lift your legs by your ankles, lean back slightly, and gently move them from side to side. Stop right away if it hurts. You can also do something similar by yourself. Lie on your back with your arms stretched out sideways. Bring one foot as far across the other leg as it'll go. This gives a good stretch to your spine and often helps one-sided pain.**

HOW AND WHERE?

People in orthopedic wards in hospitals are sometimes treated with traction, when weights are attached to the pelvis or legs for long periods. But traction can be applied for short periods, say 15–20 minutes, to people who are not bedridden. This might be done during visits to a treatment clinic such as a physiotherapy department. Then the period of treatment will be stretched out, probably being repeated up to 3 times per week for several weeks.

Nowadays, most traction is done in the physiotherapy outpatient clinic. In the past, when people were stuck in the hospital having long periods of traction, their muscles wasted. Then, when they did finally get off the traction and out of bed, their muscles were so weak they couldn't keep their spine stable, and they lost the benefits from the treatment.

Outpatient traction is usually applied electronically. You lie on the treatment table. The traction machine (note: machine, not engine!) is attached to the strap around your pelvis by a rope. The machine is then adjusted to the correct weight for you, depending on your problem and body size. Some therapists apply a constant weight for the whole 20 minutes or so of the treatment session; others use intermittent traction. In this case, the traction will pull at its maximum for about 30 seconds, followed by a comparative rest period of half-pull power for around 10 seconds. This on–almost-off pattern is continued for the length of the session.

A good traction table splits in the middle. As the weight is applied, the lower section of the table moves on rollers to accommodate the tension that is applied to your back. This means that not so much weight is needed to actually pull on your spine, as the friction of the maneuver is reduced.

Traction can be used on its own or alongside other methods of treatment, such as electrical therapies (see IDEA 17, *It's electric*) or massage treatments, as in IDEA 13, *Hands on*.

Try another idea...

THE GRAVITY OF THE SITUATION

You can apply gentle traction to yourself at home, taking care not to harm your back. Hanging by both of your arms from a door or other strong, tall structure could give temporary relief from your back pain. Place a cloth over the door, near the hinges. (Pulling the door off and wrestling with it on your knees isn't gonna do you much good.) Grip the top of the door over the cloth with your hands and slowly lift your body off the ground.

Alternatively, place two upright chairs near enough together that you can sit on the floor between them with an elbow and forearm on each seat. Gently lift your butt off the ground and let your body hang.

"To go beyond is as wrong as to fall short."
ENGLISH PROVERB

Defining idea...

CAN TRACTION DO HARM?

Traction can give you increased pain if the outer layer of the nerve is stuck to the tissue around it through inflammation. Then, when the weights pull on the spine, you will yelp. Sometimes the benefits you gain during traction are lost by the time you have struggled off the bed. But then, you're not in any condition to complain, are you?

WHEN DOES TRACTION HELP?

If you have an arthritic spine, traction might help. The stretching movements of the traction may well help if you've been immobile.

With an intervertebral disc problem, where the center of the disc is bulging but has not actually slipped out between the two vertebrae, relieving the pressure on it by using traction can help it settle back into place.

How did it go?

Q **My mother's pain seemed worse after having traction to her spine—can that happen?**

A *If your therapist has made a wrong diagnosis and you actually have a serious condition, such as cancer affecting your spine or thin bones from osteoporosis, traction might do your spine harm. If she is still suffering, suggest that your mother see her doctor at the earliest convenience.*

Q **My pain is worse when I lie flat. Will traction make this worse?**

A *No. Usually the pain from lying flat is caused by your back forming an arch. To avoid this, the therapist will put your legs on a cushion or stool during treatment to keep your back straight. In fact, you should try this at home anyway—you never know, it might mean you won't need traction after all.*

17

It's electric

Get wired up and try electrical therapy. Charge your therapist to get on with it; there'll be no shocks. And if it works, you'll have the impulse to repeat it again and again.

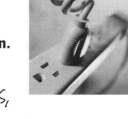

Therapy can be all about electrodes, wires, and machines. Forget alternative therapies, try alternating currents instead.

Electrical therapies speed up the healing process and relieve back pain. Not every therapist will be able to provide every electrical therapy—that'll depend on what machines they've got and what training they've had. We don't know for sure which electrical therapies work best for what conditions, or how well they work. Different doctors and therapists have their own views and preferences—so you may get conflicting advice if you consult different practitioners.

LET'S HEAR IT FOR ULTRASOUND

Ultrasound works by causing a reaction in the body's tissues that stimulates a healing response. The high-frequency sound waves that are ultrasound affect the healing process and reduce your pain. It's useful for helping the soft tissues surrounding the spine, where there's a lot of muscle spasm and general inflammation. Therapy is limited by the sound waves bouncing off the bone and being reflected back.

Here's an idea for you... **Try using a TENS machine to control your back pain instead of drugs. You can buy this device by mail order, via specialist shops and pharmacists, or directly from the manufacturer. Attaching the TENS machine to a belt underneath your clothing will render it invisible—and you can walk about normally.**

Your physiotherapist, osteopath, or chiropractor may offer you ultrasound. They'll apply gel to the treatment head of the ultrasound machine and move that slowly over the skin of your back or other affected areas of your body for a few minutes. The gel prevents there being gaps between the contours of your body and the metal treatment head. There's no heat from the machine and the application is usually painless—though sometimes, pain can be increased for a few hours afterward. You'll usually have a few treatment sessions, often once or twice a week—unless you're a world famous sports star, in which case you'll get it twice a day. Sometimes you get good pain relief after just one session.

SHORT-WAVE DIATHERMY CAN WORK

This electrical treatment creates an electromagnetic field in the body's tissues that alternates direction rapidly and can produce heat. It's usually given in a pulsed form so that the heating effect doesn't occur. Its effect comes from an alteration in the charges on cell membranes that reduces inflammation and re-establishes normality in your body's tissues.

Interferential therapy is given as two currents of varying frequency passed through the body's tissues. Stimulating those tissues increases the blood flow through the treated area, resulting in reduced pain. The electrodes may be either strapped onto your skin or attached by a vacuum extraction device. If you're taking warfarin pills to thin your blood, creating the vacuum may bruise your skin, so interferential therapy won't be right for you.

TRANSCUTANEOUS ELECTRICAL NERVE STIMULATION (TENS)

TENS usually involves two electrodes being placed on your skin on either side of the affected area, which is easy enough to do yourself. The electrodes are flexible pads connected to the TENS machine by thin wires, through which an electrical pulse is passed. The settings can be varied. A low intensity with a high-frequency pulse avoids triggering muscle contractions. A low-frequency option comparable to acupuncture can be delivered at high intensity so that it triggers visible muscle contractions. When the spinal cord is bombarded with impulses from the TENS machine, it's distracted from transmitting the pain signals from the affected painful area to your brain. TENS relieves symptoms rather than influences the speed of recovery from either acute or chronic lower back pain—an hour of use can give several hours of relief afterward.

LASER THERAPY

Laser therapy uses light waves to stimulate healing in soft tissues. It has a similar effect to ultrasound. Both you and the practitioner will have to use protective eyewear.

ELECTROMYOGRAPHIC BIOFEEDBACK

You can learn to control the tension in your muscles by receiving feedback on their electrical activity. The feedback is given as a noise or picture. Electromyographic biofeedback for lower back pain aims to relax the paraspinal muscles running along your spine.

Laser therapy can be used on acupuncture points instead of needles to relieve your pain. For more on acupuncture, see **IDEA 19, *A jab well done.***

Try another idea...

"I'm in charge."
BRUCE FORSYTH

Defining idea...

77

How did it go?

Q   Are there any no-nos for trying out electrical therapies?

A   *You shouldn't have electrical treatments (except a TENS machine) if you're pregnant or have cancer. They can upset a hearing aid or heart pacemaker, so tell your therapist in advance, don't just keel over. Some even interfere with cell phones and electric locks on car key rings—so remove your keys from your pocket or you'll have to walk home after your treatment.*

Q   I have a pacemaker—can I use a TENS machine?

A   *Sorry, you can't use a TENS machine if you have a pacemaker. You also shouldn't use a TENS machine while you're driving a car or operating machinery. Women in the first three months of pregnancy should not place the TENS electrodes on their torso or pelvis in case it harms the developing baby, although I'd relent later in your pregnancy. I'd also warn that TENS should not be put over any sensitive or broken skin, your heart, or the front of your neck.*

18
Lie down and take it

It pays to see a specialist when you're racked with back pain. You'll give a thumbs-up to the hands-on techniques of your chiropractor or osteopath.

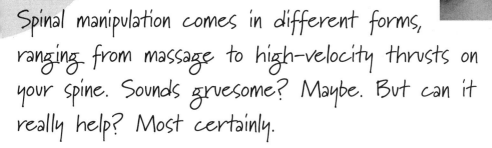

Spinal manipulation comes in different forms, ranging from massage to high-velocity thrusts on your spine. Sounds gruesome? Maybe. But can it really help? Most certainly.

Manipulation seems to be most effective in people with acute lower back pain without leg pain or pinched nerves. It increases the range of movement of your spine. Sometimes pain can be worse after manipulation, though usually only in the short term. If it persists, then manipulation is not for you and you should seek help elsewhere.

CHIROPRACTIC

Chiropractic manipulation can help with chronic or severe back pain. Going to consult a chiropractor for your back pain will get you a full assessment, involving

Here's an idea for you... **Get your money's worth by asking the chiropractor or osteopath to look at other joints that are troubling you, too. Your chiropractor could help with neck and shoulder problems, sports injuries, whiplash, and repetitive strain injuries. Your osteopath may spot that you're putting undue stress on your back from the kind of job you do, the sports you play, or the type of life you lead. They'll both advise you how to prevent your back problems from recurring.**

the diagnosis, treatment, and prevention of your back pain. Chiropractors believe that the healthiness of your spine influences the health of your whole body. They'll ask for any personal details that are relevant—such as any other illnesses or injuries you've had, what kind of work you do, what kind of chairs you sit in or bed you sleep on.

Chiropractors use their hands, rather than electrical equipment, to manipulate or adjust your spine. They push, pull, and lever muscle against bone. They'll give you general advice, such as avoiding bed rest, increasing your exercise, leading a healthy lifestyle, and discuss any psychological barriers to your recovery.

WHAT DOES CHIROPRACTIC TREATMENT ENTAIL?

You'll undress to your underclothes (socks optional), so that the chiropractor can examine the range of movements of your spine. The chiropractor may arrange X-rays of your back to help with the diagnosis and rule out any underlying diseases. You'll then lie down on a table so that the chiropractor can manipulate your vertebrae by sharp thrusts with his hands on your spine. The chiropractor uses manipulation to increase flexibility if your spine is too stiff. If he thinks your back ligaments are too slack, he'll free nearby joints that may have become stiff from compensating for the misalignment. He'll also suggest exercises for strengthening and stabilizing your back muscles. Treatments last about 15 minutes and may be one of a series over a few weeks.

You'll probably be given advice about posture and sets of exercises to do at home in between treatment sessions. Some chiropractors go for active rehabilitation, which involves fitness and endurance programs tailored to your ability.

If you don't want treatment that's too vigorous, maybe you should think about massage. The various techniques in IDEA 13, *Hands on*, will help with muscle stiffness, too.

Try another idea...

HOW DO YOU FIND A CHIROPRACTOR YOU CAN TRUST?

In the United States, chiropractors complete a four-year post-college degree, which covers the use of manipulative treatment, diagnosis of the various conditions causing back pain, and use of X-rays. The American Chiropractic Association (www.amerchiro.org) maintains listings of board certified chiropractors.

MAKE NO BONES ABOUT IT—OSTEOPATHY CAN HELP

Osteopaths are trained to recognize and treat many causes of pain. They believe that for true health, physical, social, and mental well-being are linked. Correcting the body's structure improves its function and promotes self-healing. An osteopath uses his hands to diagnose the problem, examining your spine when you're at rest and watching as you move your back around in sitting, standing, and walking. He'll look at the rest of your body, too, as a problem in one area of your body can effect another part.

"The hand that gives, gathers."
ENGLISH PROVERB

Defining idea...

Defining idea...

"Ready money works great cures."
FRENCH PROVERB

Osteopathy uses your arms and legs as long levers or fulcrums for twisting and bending your body. Osteopaths use their hands to stretch soft tissues and mobilize joints through rhythmic, passive movements and high-velocity thrust techniques, to improve your mobility and range of joint movement. This should reduce the strain on your other joints and thereby improve your general mobility and health. An osteopathy treatment is often accompanied by an audible "click." Despite the sound effects, osteopathy is usually painless.

Q   **Is it true that manipulation is dangerous if you have cancer? My mother has bone cancer, and her back pain is getting her down.**

How did it go?

A   *Manipulation should not be used in pregnant women or in patients with cancer, severe or progressive neurological symptoms, osteoporosis, where the back pain is originating from other parts of the body than the spine, or ankylosing spondylitis, as it might potentially cause a worsening of the symptoms or even a fracture if the manipulated spine is osteoporotic. However, there are few risks from manipulation for lower back pain, provided that the patients are selected and assessed properly and it's carried out by a trained practitioner. Then there's probably only a one in a million chance of manipulation doing harm. In fact, the X-rays that the practitioners order may be more harmful than the actual treatment itself.*

Q   **How do I choose which type of manipulation to try since it's so costly?**

A   *It's impossible to predict exactly who will respond and when, or what kind of manipulation is most effective in relieving pain or increasing spinal movement. Physiotherapists, osteopaths, chiropractors, and some medical practitioners obviously favor their own speciality's way of performing manipulation. And if you're paying for your treatment, you might persuade yourself that it works better than something you get free from your health insurance! So unless somebody's recommended one treatment over another, flip a coin!*

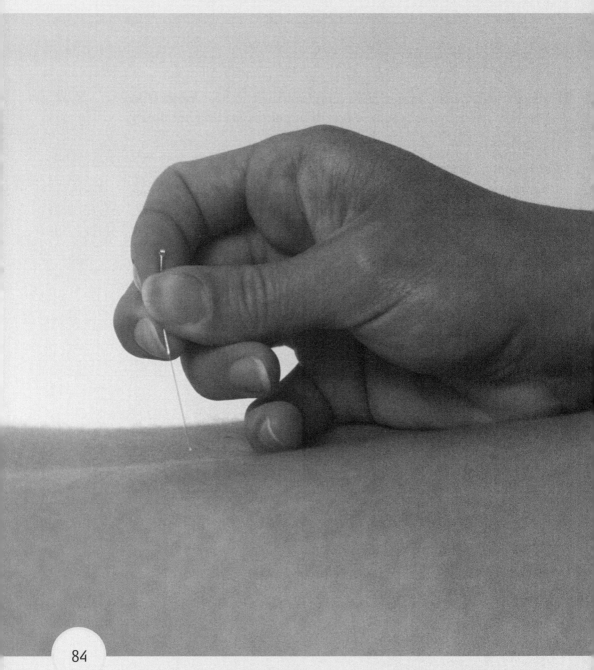

19

A jab well done

You might think you were in enough pain already without some stranger using you as a pincushion. Still, it's been good enough for the Chinese for more than 3,000 years, so why not give acupuncture a try?

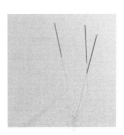

Acupuncture considers the whole body rather than concentrating solely on specific symptoms, as Western medicine tends to do. This holistic approach is all you'll "needle."

Acupuncture originated in China and has been practiced for more than 3000 years. Acupuncture points run along "meridian" channels. Needles are inserted into specific designated points on the body relating to particular sites of pain suffered by the patient or client. Stimulation from the needle points redirects channels of energy beneath the skin to restore the body's energy levels (called *qi* or *chi*) and create "harmony" in your normal bodily functions.

WHAT'S THE POINT?

Don't worry about ending up looking like a hedgehog. The usual Western approach is to insert a few fine needles (perhaps three or four) for around 20 minutes or so. With the Chinese approach, needles may be left in for up to an hour. The

Here's an idea for you...

You can get a similar effect to acupuncture through acupoint stimulation. You can stimulate your own acupuncture points with an electric stimulator—a device shaped like a fat pen with a metal tip. These are available from some pharmacies or through mail order.

practitioner may rotate the needles in the skin to re-stimulate the acupuncture point. Different acupuncturists use different techniques. They vary as to the sites of the body, lengths of time needles are left in, and whether they attach small electric currents to the needles (electroacupuncture) or use heated herbs (*moxa*) to warm them. That's a lot of choice, but don't let that become a sticking point. Disposable needles are usually used, as they are reasonably cheap. Otherwise, the needles should be carefully sterilized, to avoid the spread of transmissible diseases like AIDS or hepatitis.

Acupressure is another approach. This entails the application of finger pressure to acupuncture sites. It's thought not to be as powerful as using needles, and the benefits may be more like those from deep massage. The acupressure is sometimes applied through fixing a plant seed on the skin, or using a pencil point or magnetic balls.

Did you know? Fewer side effects are associated with acupuncture than with prescribed painkillers.

WHO ARE THE ACUPUNCTURISTS?

Take care to choose an acupuncturist with the right qualifications, because licensing requirements vary from state to state. In the United States, licensed acupuncturists bear the letters L. Ac. after their name. Ask the acupuncturist when you book your appointment how and where they trained. Some are doctors and therapists who have just learned to do acupuncture as a sideline; others are pure acupuncturists. Some have spent time in China, where acupuncture is a routine method of providing pain relief and treating many other conditions, learning and practicing their techniques according to the Chinese culture.

Don't stick to acupuncture as your sole treatment—try reflexology. See IDEA 23, *Your sparking zones.*

Try another idea...

SO HOW DOES IT WORK?

It's worthwhile going under the needle. There is plenty of research to show that acupuncture can lessen your back pain and help you to be more active if you suffer from chronic lower back pain.

Energy flows around your body and keeps everything healthy. If anything is wrong with you, then the energy flow is compromised and the blockage needs to be cleared. The lack of health might be a pain in your back or elsewhere, but it could also be inflammation, sickness, or psychological problems. Acupuncture restores the situation to normal by getting energy to flow through the affected areas. Applying needles to the body creates small electrical currents and helps energy to flow along the meridian channels into which the acupuncture needles have been inserted.

"Tetigisti acu *(Latin translation: "You've hit the point")."*
PLAUTUS

Defining idea...

EAR, EAR

Particular points on your body affect areas quite distant from them or stimulate parts of the brain to control pain. (This has been verified by research.) For example, the whole body is represented topographically on the ear. If an area of the body needs treatment, then the corresponding point on the ear will become sensitive. These points can be found by using an electrical point-finder or a blunt needle handle. Some acupuncturists then use these points on the ear to effect treatment.

How did it go?

Q   My acupuncturist said I need ten sessions—but it's expensive. Is there an alternative?

A   How many treatment sessions you will need depends on your response to your first few acupuncture sessions and your practitioner's usual practice. You could get a second opinion, or ask your acupuncturist straight out if you can get by with fewer visits. If she's adamant that only ten will do the trick, either leave the course early and see if you can get by or decide which is the most important—a happy back or a happy wallet.

Q   I have had acupuncture recently to relax me because I was stressed. My friend has used it for pregnancy sickness and another friend for back pain. How can it work for all these problems? Are we being had?

A   There is research to show that acupuncture works in animals—which shows that you don't need to believe in it to know that it works. More and more research is being carried out that shows acupuncture works for all sorts of different conditions in humans, too, like those you've mentioned here.

20

At the core of the matter

Whether you sit at a desk all day or spend most of your time doing heavy work, you need core strength. With Pilates you can build up the muscles of your spine.

Pilates exercises will help you maintain a healthy back through good movements and good posture. Pilates won't help you fly, but it will change the way you look, feel, and move.

Find a trained teacher in Pilates and join a class, or go to a physiotherapist, chiropractor, or osteopath who can take you through a Pilates program. Pilates exercises are of increasing difficulty. You must be careful not to attempt anything too difficult when you're just starting out: You will need to build up your stamina to improve your endurance first. With Pilates, you figure out for yourself what's the best possible combination of exercises for you and chop and change accordingly.

GOING THE PILATES WAY

You start by taking time to relax, to prepare your body and mind for your exercise session. You'll concentrate on the movements that you make, being really aware of your body and that you're ready to exercise. You'll focus on your breathing and how

89

Here's an idea for you...

Some exercises can be practiced anywhere. Sliding down a wall, for instance, can be done even when space is limited, such as in an office or even on board an airplane. Stand with your back to the wall and your feet about 6 inches away from it, parallel to and the same width apart as your hips. Lean back against the wall and stand comfortably. Breathe in, lengthening your spine. Then breathe out, contracting your pelvic and abdominal muscles. Now bend your knees and slide about 12 inches down the wall, keeping your tailbone in contact with the wall. Don't take your butt below knee level. Keep your heels on the floor with your feet flat and parallel throughout. Breathe in as you slide back up trying to keep the base of your spine lengthened as far as possible. Repeat up to 8 times, unless it hurts.

it feels to breathe right. As you breathe out you'll pull your muscles up and in from your pelvis and abdomen. All this helps to create a strong, central spine. Then you'll be ready to undertake Pilates exercises in a rhythmic, smooth way, moving without strain or stress to your back or the rest of your body.

EXERCISING

There are beginner's exercises to improve the stability of your lumbar spine. With Pilates, you're aiming to be able to contract the muscles of your pelvic floor at the same time as hollowing your lower abdominal muscles, drawing them back toward your spine. The pelvic floor comprises the muscles of the urethra in men and of the vagina in women. Once you've learned how to contract these sets of muscles, you'll learn to do so in lots of different positions, not just sitting in a chair. This might be kneeling on all fours on the floor, lying prone on your stomach, or lying in the relaxation position on your back, with your knees bent up and your feet flat on the ground.

With this skill on hand, Pilates exercises can help you to align your spine centrally. They are designed to isolate and work on the deep stabilizing muscles of your pelvis and spine, as well as your other bones and joints. They help you move individual segments of your spine safely.

Pilates exercises can really help you get your pelvic and abdominal muscles ready for pregnancy. See IDEA 43, *Mom's the word*, for more on this.

Try another idea...

In a healthy back, all the interlinking vertebrae work together, like in a bicycle chain. If one area of your back becomes stiff or damaged, it effects the neighboring vertebrae, which may change their structure and movement to compensate for the problem one. This puts strain on your back. Many Pilates exercises work toward promoting the flexibility and stability of your spine. They include spine curls, hip flexor stretches, shoulder drops, neck rolls and chin tucks, arm openings, side rolls of your trunk, side reaches, and many others.

You need to create the right environment for doing Pilates. Find a time and a place where you're not hassled by telephone calls or children's demands. Get a padded mat to exercise on, with plenty of room around, and wear loose, light clothing. Go barefoot so you're more aware of your body's movements. Do remember that if you've got a back problem, such as a slipped disc, you should take advice from a trained Pilates practitioner before attempting any of the exercises.

"Be prepared."
BOY SCOUT MOTTO

Defining idea...

How did
it go? **Q** **My pelvic floor is now so well honed it has its own six-pack. How long until I can try more advanced exercises?**

A *Once you've mastered the beginner's exercises you can move on to intermediate and then advanced exercises to build on your increasingly stable and strong spine. These exercises can be individualized for people doing specific jobs at work.*

Q **Really? So how does Pilates help people in different types of jobs?**

A *Pilates exercises can counter the effects of sitting at a desk, and strengthen your back to cope with any repetitive movements in your everyday work. Exercises to keep lengthening and maintaining the curves of your spine can be done while driving long distances. For manual workers, Pilates exercises help by developing deep postural muscles and increasing your awareness of moving correctly. Sportsmen and women use Pilates to establish a strong postural base upon which they can build muscles for the particular techniques needed in their sports. If the sport requires unilateral strength, such as with golf, that places repetitive strain on the lumbar vertebrae, which Pilates exercises can help to counterbalance. Singers and actors are helped by breathing exercises, with their voice projection and improving their endurance in standing around at rehearsals. Musicians are helped by core Pilates exercises and ones specifically for their hands and fingers. There ain't nothin' Pilates can't do!*

21

Little and large

A little help from your friends, the homeopaths, can have a large benefit. Your back pain may subside little by little with homeopathic remedies.

Like cures like. Substances that in large doses will cause the symptoms of an illness can be used in minute quantities to relieve those same symptoms.

HOMEOPATHY WORKS

It works by stimulating your body's capacity to heal itself. You'll fight your disease or health problem after causing an initial aggravation of the problem. So you can only expect homeopathic medicine to cure your health problems when it's possible that your body can repair itself. For more serious conditions, like cancer, homeopathic remedies can only help lessen the symptoms.

You can buy homeopathic treatments from shops and pharmacies, or they can be prescribed by homeopathic practitioners. Some are branded medicines and others are flower remedies. They can help coughs and colds, digestive complaints, skin conditions, and joint pains.

Here's an idea for you... **Try a homeopathic injection for your back. Some homeopathic practitioners use formica (the sting of ants) and acus mold (the sting of honeybees) for injections into joints as an alternative to steroid injections. The sting is diluted many times, but may still trigger a reaction to the venom to stimulate a healing effect.**

GET YOUR ENERGY MEDICINE

Homeopathic medicine is tailored to your healing capacity and immune response. The remedies are derived from natural sources, such as a plant, mineral, or animal secretion. Plants include belladonna (the deadly nightshade), arnica, and chamomile; minerals include mercury and sulphur; and animal products include squid ink and snake venom. The remedies are prepared by a repeated process of dilution and violent shaking. The more times the process is repeated, the more potent the homeopathic remedy is thought to be. As a result, there's very little active ingredient present. This makes some people wonder if homeopathic remedies have any effect at all, other than that because you're told it's a remedy it does actually make you feel better. Other people swear that even very dilute homeopathic medicines act on people's biological function at the cellular level.

Homeopathic medicines with a wide spectrum of activity are called *polychrests*; while *complex* remedies are a mixture of medicines usually with specific uses. Homeopathic remedies may be given as pills, granules, or powders, or in liquid form. They're dissolved in your mouth rather than swallowed, and you're advised not to take food or drink for 15 minutes or so before or after taking a remedy.

The numbers after the names indicate the extent of dilution; 6c is generally recommended for ailments that have developed over a long period of time, whereas the stronger 30c is generally used for acute conditions. Potentially toxic concentrations of some homeopathic drugs have been described, and there are occasional allergic reactions.

HOMEOPATHIC REMEDIES FOR BACK PAIN

There are more than 2,000 substances used by homeopaths to treat diseases. Examples of homeopathic medicines that are recommended for various forms of back pain include: acetic acid, bryonia, gnaphalium, ledum, and sepia. A homeopathic practitioner will specify the type of treatment that is appropriate for different sites and descriptions of pain and weakness, and prescribe treatment until improvement occurs. Side effects are more likely with the more concentrated doses, and include: laxative (e.g., bryonia), gastric irritant or abortion (e.g., ledum), and heart failure (e.g., aconite).

To understand the thinking behind complementary medicine, look back at IDEA 12, *What's the alternative?*

Try another idea...

TAKING YOUR MEDICINE

The homeopath will want to know all about you, as each person is treated uniquely. He'll want to gauge your susceptibility to disease, and how you're affected by your condition—emotionally and physically. Tell him about anything you've had wrong with you in the past, all about your symptoms and how they vary with what you do or the time of the year, and so on.

The homeopath will then match the right remedy with your symptoms and circumstances. He might give a different remedy to you than to somebody else with the same condition—matching it to your personal makeup. For a chronic problem,

"A little of what you fancy does you good."
ANONYMOUS

Defining idea...

he'll expect you to take the remedy for some months. He'll review your progress periodically and readjust the nature or strength of the remedy as necessary. It'll be reduced as soon as your symptoms improve, and stopped if they seem to have been aggravated or if you're better.

FINDING A HOMEOPATH YOU CAN TRUST

Training in homeopathy can vary from 40 hours for a doctor to three-year university degrees. Licensing varies state by state. Certification is available through the Council for Homeopathic Certification (www.homeopathicdirectory.com).

Q I have a sensitive stomach. Are there any adverse effects from using homeopathic medicines that I should be aware of?

How did it go?

A *Because homeopathic remedies are so dilute they are non-toxic and can be taken at all ages and during pregnancy. Most side effects of homeopathic medicines are mild and short term. You might get a brief aggravation of your symptoms—after all, that's how the homeopathic medicine basically works. You could experience headaches, tiredness, skin rash, dizziness, or diarrhea, but these type of symptoms will quickly pass (through you, in the last case).*

Q I take homeopathic medicine, so is it okay to take other drugs prescribed by my doctor as well?

A *Some homeopathic remedies can clash with the conventional drugs you get from a doctor. It's always best to check first with the doc, or tell your homeopathic practitioner what other medicines you're taking.*

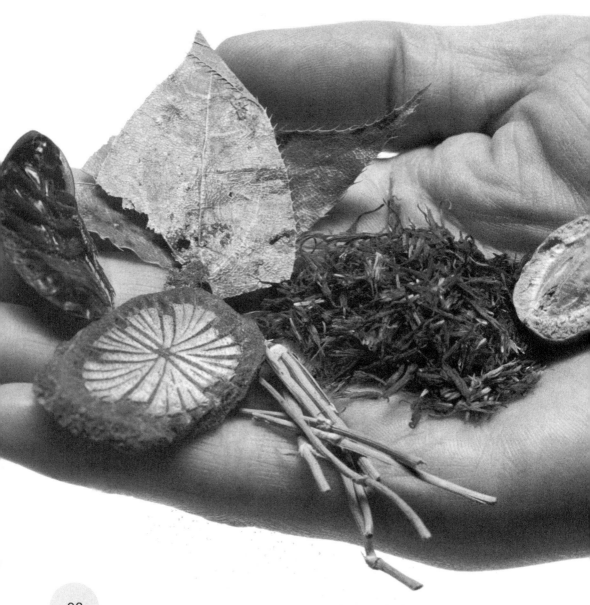

22

Find your roots

It's no surprise if you want to see whether herbal medicines work for you—it's only natural. Try an extract and you'll want much more.

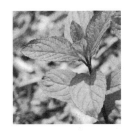

The Chinese go for yin (cooling) and yang (stimulating).

Herbal medicines are made from roots, flowers, herbs, bark, or plant extracts. The herbalist makes use of the whole plant to make up the remedy rather than using a single active ingredient from the plant, as conventional drugs do. Because they are natural, they're one of the most popular forms of complementary medicine.

HERBAL REMEDIES

Herbal medicines may be tried for a wide range of conditions, including back pain. Other common uses are for sleeplessness, listlessness, and general aches and pains. They're usually taken for generalized conditions rather than for single diseases, being thought to act on the body's systems by their anti-inflammatory or antispasmodic properties. Herbal remedies are targeted at the underlying cause of the illness to restore good health, as well as at your immediate symptoms, like back pain.

Here's an idea for you...

Don't let safety worries deter you from trying herbal medicines—just be careful. If you're buying herbal remedies from a health food store or pharmacy, read the label or ask the vendor. If you're consulting with a doctor or nurse, tell them—or better still, show them—what herbal medicines you're taking before they give you a prescription. Be ready to stop your herbals if there's likely to be a clash with your prescribed conventional treatment.

HERBAL PREPS

St. John's Wort is an extract from the shrub Hypericum. Usually given in doses from 300 to 1,000 milligrams, it works by improving any underlying anxiety and depression, rather than by having a direct effect on the source of your back pain. You may suffer side effects, such as oversensitivity to light and the formation of cataracts in your eyes. Other side effects include stomach upsets, tiredness, and restlessness. St. John's Wort can also interact with many prescribed drugs, such as contraceptives, blood thinning pills, heart pills, antidepressant drugs, and epileptic treatments. Suddenly your back pain doesn't seem so bad after all, does it?

Glucosamine sulphate is regarded as "food for cartilage." It's thought to stimulate production of cartilage components and allow rebuilding of damaged cartilage. Glucosamine is usually taken as 1.5 grams by mouth in divided doses during the day or as an injection of 400 milligrams 2–3 times per week. Side effects are few, but may include mild stomach pain, heartburn, drowsiness, diarrhea, and nausea. Research has shown that glucosamine is effective for arthritis pain, and is as effective as taking 1.2 grams (that's 6 regular tabs to you and me) per day of the non-steroidal anti-inflammatory drug ibuprofen, at least in the short term.

Red pepper extract—topical capsium—or black pepper is also known as "substance P," which is used for pains in the joints. It's taken continuously rather than as an ad-hoc treatment. Adverse reactions depend on the dose you take and how concentrated it is. They include eye symptoms, a burning pain in your nose or sneezing, cough, skin irritation, and discomfort of your stomach.

To find out more about the potential hazards from herbal medicines and conventional treatments, visit IDEA 48, *Trick or treat?*

Try another idea...

Celery seeds have been used to relieve rheumatic pains. Adverse effects include sedation and dermatitis, and they can also prompt allergic reactions. Some experts warn against taking any quantity greater than that contained in food.

Capsaicin, derived from chili peppers, is used as a cream for treating pain, especially pain after shingles, and from rheumatoid arthritis or osteoarthritis. Just be careful where you rub it.

INDIVIDUAL TO YOU

The herbalist will recommend an herbal treatment based on your current symptoms, general health and lifestyle, and previous and other illnesses. They should also ask whether you're taking any other medication—especially if prescribed by a doctor—so they can avoid any potential interactions. They'll generally make up an individual remedy for you. This may be a pill or a tincture—a concentrated solution of herbs extracted in water and alcohol. Alternatively, you might be given raw herbs to boil in water and drink as tea.

Defining
idea...

"Formerly when religion was strong and science weak, men mistook magic for medicine. Now when science is strong and religion weak, men mistake medicine for magic."
THOMAS SZASZ

WATCH OUT

Sometimes conventional drugs are added to seemingly herbal medicines to increase their effectiveness. If that's the case, and you're taking the same medication prescribed by your doctor, you could easily overdose. Read the fine print.

Q   Are herbal medicines regulated by the government?

How did it go?

A   *Herbal medicines are not subject to such strict controls as regulated pharmaceutical medicines—yet. Because of this, the source and quality of most herbal remedies have not been standardized. Herbal medicines have been known to be contaminated by other substances. This is rare, but there have been fatalities—for example, from kidney failure after taking contaminated herbal preparations for treating eczema.*

Q   OK. How safe are they without contaminants?

A   *Most herbal remedies prescribed by a qualified and experienced herbalist are safe. But just because herbal medicines are "natural" doesn't mean that they're necessarily safe, and some are highly toxic. They can have adverse effects such as diarrhea or anemia, or can worsen other diseases such as schizophrenia. They may interact with medication prescribed by a doctor or bought over the counter. This could trigger side effects or even heighten the effect of the conventional drug you've been prescribed. For instance, if you suffer from epilepsy and took evening primrose oil alongside your anticonvulsant treatment, you'd be more likely to have epileptic fits.*

Q   How do I find an herbalist I can trust?

A   *Contact your regional herbal association. Beware the inadequately qualified herbalist who gives you an unusual combination of herbs which might clash when put together and make you unwell. Oranges and pinks, for example.*

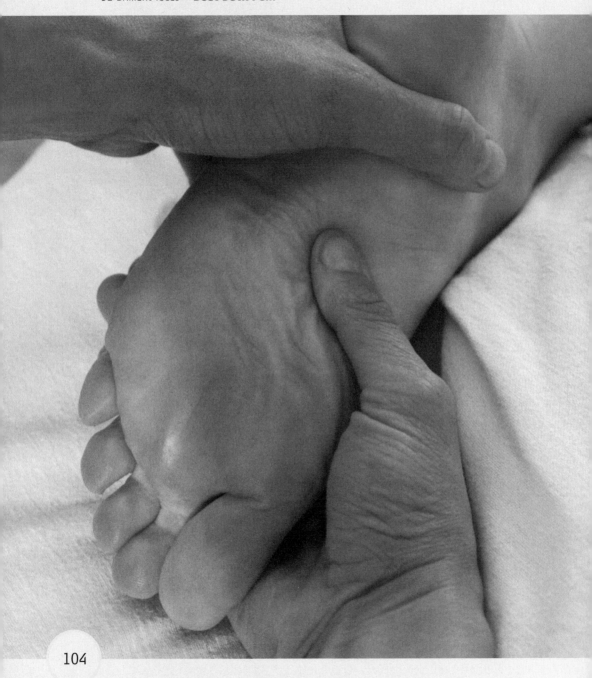

23

Your sparking zones

Mirror, mirror on my feet, can you my back pain please delete? With reflexology you'll venture into foot-charted territory to fight your pain.

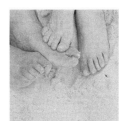

You'll have a reflex reaction as your reflexologist pressures you to encourage your body's natural healing processes.

Reflexology can help to combat the pain of osteoarthritis and sciatica. Reflexing is a form of therapeutic massage given to areas of the hands and feet to produce specific beneficial effects in other parts of your body. The underside of the foot, or palm of the hand, is like a chart of your body. Specific reflex points on your hands and feet correspond to certain parts of your body: bones, muscles, organs, glands, circulation, and nerve pathways. The reflexologist sees illness as the result of an energy imbalance in specific organs or structures of your body, for instance, your spine. The imbalance is reflected in the corresponding area of the soles of your feet—so treat the foot and the corresponding organ or structure benefits.

HOW THE ZONES WORK OUT

A reflexologist sees your body as being divided into ten equal vertical zones running the length of your body, from the top of the head to the tips of the toes. Every zone ends with a finger or toe. Each has reflex points linked with corresponding areas of

Here's an idea for you...

Some reflexologists use a vacuum pump and suction kit, called a vacuflex, to identify problem areas. You wear a special pair of boots from which all the air is pumped to vac-pac your feet. This has the effect of stimulating all your reflex points at the same time. When the boots are removed soon afterward, discolored areas indicate the points of imbalance in your body. The reflexologist then uses small suction pads to stimulate the appropriate reflex points.

the body. The right foot relates to the right side of the body, and likewise the left. The zone thought to correspond with your spine runs along the inside edge of the big toe and onto the inside edge of the rest of your foot, while that linked to the sciatic nerve is on the sole of your foot close to your heel.

As well as applying pressure to reflex points on your feet, your reflexologist will give you a general foot massage. Reflexology can give you the generalized benefits of relaxation and general well-being, and it can help reduce anxiety, stress, and muscular tension. After a session you'll be glowing.

USING REFLEXOLOGY TO BEAT BACK PAIN

A course of treatment usually comprises 6–8 sessions, each lasting 45 minutes to an hour. Before starting, the reflexologist will ask you about your symptoms and lifestyle, and what else you've had wrong with you in the past. She'll then examine the soles of your feet and the palms of your hands while you stretch out in a special chair. She may start the treatment by dusting your feet with talcum powder and giving them a gentle massage—a great icebreaker, and one that enables her to locate any tender areas at the same time. She'll then apply pressure to points on your feet and hands with her thumbs and fingers, in a caterpillar-like movement. Feet are worked on more often than hands, as they're larger and more sensitive. The tender areas will usually become less painful as the massaging treatment

continues. Some reflexologists use herbal
ointment or oil at the end of a treatment to
stimulate your circulation, help you relax, and
make you want to return for more!

Why not try reflexology out on yourself? For other methods of self-help, see IDEA 3, *Help yourself*.

Try another idea...

Tender or painful areas indicate a blockage or depletion of energy. By applying
finger and thumb pressure, the practitioner releases tension and unblocks
previously stuck energy. Massaging both of your feet in this way treats both sides of
your body. Reflexologists explain the process as mechanically breaking down
crystalline deposits of uric acid or calcium. These are then carried away by the
bloodstream and eliminated from your body as a form of detoxification. This is the
cleansing response, and you might get side effects such as headaches, sweating,
or diarrhea.

After your reflexology session you should feel relaxed and may crave sleep. You
might experience warmth in the injured area of your back. Hopefully it will have
relieved you of some of your back pain and loosened any stiffness.

"There's language in her eye, her cheek, her lip; Nay, her foot speaks."
WILLIAM SHAKESPEARE

Defining idea...

How did
it go?

Q **Reflexology does help me, but when my practitioner massages my feet, it sometimes feels like I'm being cut by glass. Why?**

A *This feeling of nails or glass digging in during massage is well recognized with reflexology. Reflexologists explain this as areas of grittiness developing in the parts of the feet that correspond with distant parts of the body that are affected by ill-health problems, though it could just be sand in the oil.*

Q **I get athlete's foot from time to time. Is it still okay to have reflexology?**

A *You're better not having reflexology when you have an infected rash on your hands or feet—it might spread, and the rash could get worse from the friction of the treatment. And spare a thought for the poor reflexologist! You should also avoid reflexology if you have a bleeding disorder or are taking the blood-thinning medication warfarin, as you could suffer internal bleeding and severe bruising.*

Q **My feet are hideous. I'm ashamed to show them in public. Can I do reflexology by myself in the dark?**

A *Certainly—light has no effect. Sit on a chair or cross-legged on the floor or bed, with cushions behind your back. Copy the techniques and sequence that a professional reflexologist uses by reading up on it or mirroring previous treatments you've had. It's unlikely to be as effective as consulting a full-blown reflexologist, but it should give you some pain relief.*

24

Just a suggestion

"You will not have back pain when you wake up. You will not have back pain when you wake up. You will not..."

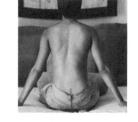

One in ten people are easy to hypnotize and the same number are resistant. Hypnosis isn't a cure. But it might help you to help yourself.

Hypnosis is that mental state where you're so deeply relaxed that you'll be open to suggestion and suspend your critical faculties. Hypnotherapists use hypnosis to help ease pain, especially persistent pain. And they use it to help people with stress, anxiety, phobias, and depression. Some people find hypnotherapy helpful in overcoming addictions like smoking. Sometimes it helps chronic illnesses like asthma or irritable bowel syndrome. Although you'll want to try it for your back pain, consider a multisymptom session if you suffer from one or more of these other conditions—they could be linked.

WHAT DO HYPNOTHERAPISTS DO?

The hypnotherapist will generally see you in a consulting room—somewhere quiet, fairly dark, and private (unless you've been dragged up onstage in a show, in which case expect lights and a little razzmatazz!). The session may last as long as an hour.

Here's an idea for you... **If you've had a few successful sessions with a hypnotist, you're probably ready to try self-hypnosis. You can be given a suggestion while you're under that will enable you to induce self-hypnosis after the treatment course has finished. With practice, you should be able to relax at will and use it to help control your back pain. Even if it doesn't lessen the actual intensity of the pain, it'll help you cope with it.**

You'll sit in a comfortable armchair, where you can lean back and relax. The hypnotherapist will probably be sitting near to you without a desk or anything between you both. She'll start off by asking all about your backache or other problems, and what other approaches you've tried. You'll need to trust the hypnotherapist and feel safe in order to relax into the hypnotic state.

Once the therapist has induced a deeply relaxed state by hypnosis, she'll make therapeutic suggestions to change your behavior or relieve your symptoms. This hypnotic trance is a state between waking and sleeping. You can be aware of everything going on around you, but at the same time feel that you're completely detached from it. You can end the trance any time you want to—you're not powerless.

Hypnotherapists have different techniques for inducing a hypnotic trance. You may be led to imagine that you're drifting comfortably away, picturing yourself in a tranquil setting, such as in an idyllic countryside scene. Your eyelids may feel heavy and your eyes gradually close.

Defining idea...

"If you want life to be more rewarding, you have to change the way you think."
OPRAH WINFREY

The sort of suggestions the hypnotherapist will make will be for you to control the level of your back pain like, say, turning down the volume control on a radio. Or she may suggest that pain is not a problem for you, so that after your hypnosis session it no longer dominates your life. Although you're open to suggestion, the hypnotherapist won't be able to make you do something you don't want to do.

Afterward, you may not remember what happened to you or what suggestions were planted.

If you've become disabled by back pain, then IDEA 50, *Living as a different you*, will help you keep your disability in proportion.

Try another idea...

AUTOGENIC TRAINING

This technique draws heavily from both hypnosis and yoga. Almost anyone can learn autogenic training by reading a self-help book and it can be mastered in only a few weeks. With autogenic training you focus on experiencing physical sensations, such as warmth and heaviness, in different parts of your body. You'll develop a sequence of very specific auto-suggestive formulas that you repeat in a specific pattern and formulized resolutions that you repeat up to thirty times. This process helps you cultivate pleasant sensations to outweigh painful stimuli.

FINDING A HYPNOTHERAPIST YOU CAN TRUST

You need to find someone you can trust—otherwise you'll be in a very vulnerable position when under. You need to be confident that the hypnotist is planting positive and helpful suggestions in your mind, rather than negative or playful ones. A few doctors, dentists, and psychologists are trained in hypnotherapy, too. Some provide hypnotherapy alongside conventional treatments, whereas others offer it on a private basis. There are also a lot of non-medically qualified hypnotherapists.

"We are all in a post-hypnotic trance induced in early infancy."
R. D. LAING

Defining idea...

111

How did it go?

Q   I tried hypnosis once in the past but had difficulty relaxing into a hypnotic state. Any tips?

A   *Imagine yourself in a tranquil setting. Practice this at home before you go for your session. Think of a particular setting you'll be able to recall easily at the hypnotism session, even when you're feeling nervous. For someone without much imagination, the hypnotherapist may get them to hold a coin in their hand. They're asked to concentrate on it, while they are talked into the hypnotic state. When the coin drops, the person's eyes will close and their body will relax.*

Q   I want to try hypnosis for my back pain, but I've had a checkered life and don't want the hypnosis to dredge up my past. What do you think I should do?

A   *Hypnosis can sometimes reawaken memories of something traumatic that you'd rather stay buried. If you're upset or have mental health problems, then you're better avoiding hypnosis. And certainly avoid it in the presence of a police officer.*

25

Let's put you in the picture

Camera. Action. Take 1. Your back is in agony, jobs are piling up, friends are bored with your moaning. Now... Take 25. You're in the gym, you're on an active vacation, laughing with your family. Figure out what it takes to get there.

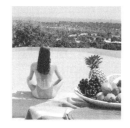

Visualization focuses on your internal experience of memories, dreams, fantasies, and visions. Visual imagery is not just about conjuring up that vision you want, but the needs of all of your senses.

Visualization can be a powerful way of counteracting painful stimuli by imposing images of you taking control of your pain, so that you're more comfortable. With visualization your mind is a videotape that you can stop, erase parts of, re-record, and so on. However, you'll want to feel that what you record on the tape is your decision and under your control, and not dictated by other people. Visualization allows you to develop a new "groove" in your brain and to change any existing old habits.

Here's an idea for you...

Visualize your back pain. Think about your back problems and when the pain is worse. Think of what triggers it and what helps it. Imagine that there is a dial you can operate to turn the intensity of your pain up or down. Once you get that image of the dial fixed in your mind, you'll be able to increase or decrease your back pain at will. As you harness your new power, you'll be able to turn that dial right down to rock bottom, diminishing the level of your pain.

CHANGE THE PICTURE

Imagine yourself without back pain. Visualization enables you to shut out negative thoughts and feelings, and focus on what you're trying to achieve—you without pain and with a mobile back. It provides an opportunity to play out a scenario in your mind and cut out the parts you don't want. It allows you to relax and to focus, even for a short time, on a particular situation. Other creative ideas will come crowding in at that moment. These have been released from that part of your consciousness that is usually suppressed by the logical, rational, and literal part of your brain.

FEEL THAT CONTROL, POWER, AND SUCCESS

Visualization allows you to create powerful pathways in your brain and generate feelings of control, power, and success. For example, imagine you're in a meeting where everyone has gathered to hear your plans to develop a project. You can practice a speech, you can imagine meeting with the people who support you and those whom you admire, you can control access to the room. In short, you imagine yourself in control and successful. These feelings will create new pathways in your brain. The more you do this, the more the image of you at the successful meeting is embedded in your mind. And the more the image is embedded, the more easily you will be able to carry out the behavior you've visualized, triggering a positive cycle of feeling, rehearsal, and achievement.

REHEARSE YOUR LIFE

Take any situation in life where you've performed well, badly, or indifferently. What would happen if you had a second chance to live through that situation again? You'd probably do things a whole lot better. In a similar way, if you've had a chance to rehearse something first, you should do a lot better when you have to do it in reality—your mind is predisposed to acting automatically in a more effective way. Visualization cannot include everything that could occur to you, but by covering many of the options that you can foresee, you should be more relaxed and confident, and should cope well with anything unexpected when it crops up.

Visualization opens you up to perceiving things differently, almost with "different parts of your brain," bypassing your normal defenses and logical, rational thoughts. Images are powerful and can be relaxing (so long as they show you in a positive and effective way). You can do this with guided imagery, too; for example imagining you are in a pleasant place where you feel contented.

Try another idea...

Find someone who has visualized successfully and pick their brain for tips. Then read IDEA 45, *Listening in*, and see who else has advice. Then try their ideas for yourself.

Defining idea...

"Imagination is the highest kite one can fly."
LAUREN BACALL

LOOK STRAIGHT AHEAD

What to visualize first? Begin with a forward-thinking idea. Put that idea into words and pictures, then convert those into a skill or service. For example, imagine where you'd like to be with regard to your lifestyle or career in five, ten, or twenty years' time. Now work backward to see what you need to change to achieve that five, ten, or twenty year vision. If you want a certain lifestyle in five years' time, what do you have to do now to achieve it? If you wish to change your career you can use visualization and imagery to decide on the type of career you'd like, and what it will entail, in great detail.

How did it go?

Q   I'm into self-hypnosis, and visualization seems pretty much like it to me. Does it to you?

A   *Yes, it is a bit like hypnosis. Both share that relaxed state that allows the use of suggestion. But with visualization, suggestions are visual and generated by you—rather than by another person, as they are in hypnosis.*

Q   Are there any forms of relaxation I can try instead of or in addition to visual imagery?

A   *You could always try progressive relaxation. With this technique, you tense a group of muscles, such as those in one arm, hold the contraction for about 15 seconds and then release it while breathing out. You continue this approach with other muscle groups, such as those in your back. Now envision yourself in a relaxed state. You can consciously deepen and slow your breathing, making yourself relax any tension you've got as you breathe out.*

26

Get a life

Take a break—from work and at work. Get your life back in balance so you don't live to work, but work to live.

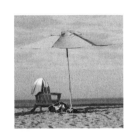

What's your ideal? A relaxed home life with your loving family? Regular time with your friends, in the gym, clubbing, or recovering afterward? Whatever it is, go for it!

Pressured board meetings and fights at home will all cause your muscles to knot up and exacerbate your back symptoms. Hunching over your PC for long hours will make your back pain worse or keep it going. So you need to get your work–life balance right.

REVIEW HOW YOU SPLIT YOUR WEEK

One of the ways to reduce the feelings of pressure is to timetable enough free time to have space for rest and relaxation to counteract the stresses and strains you're under. Try to complete work activities within your normal working hours, so that you have enough time for leisure and social chitchat. Otherwise you won't have the opportunity for personal growth outside work and may become stale.

Set a target to improve at something, like getting fit enough to run a half marathon. Set yourself a plan to crank up your fitness over a three-month period, in the gym and via a local running club.

One of the best ways to monitor whether you're managing to protect enough time for yourself is to keep a daily log of activities. Do this for a week or so. Sort your daily activities into three categories: *personal needs*, including shopping, sleeping, domestic chores, and bodily needs; *work*, including reading work-related books, reports, and papers; and *leisure*, including sport, relaxation, reading, and music.

Work out the totals for the types of activities you do per day and calculate an average over the week. Compare your daily totals with the ideal for a healthy lifestyle: 45–55 percent of your time spent on personal needs, 25–30 percent on work, and 20–25 percent on leisure. You'll find that when the proportion of your day spent on work is much more than 25 percent, it's the leisure proportion that suffers.

HOW DO YOU SPEND YOUR TIME?

Most of us feel overloaded at work these days. Are you being pulled in different directions (other than during physical therapy)? Must you call back everyone who's left messages for you? You need to have the know-how to deal with these challenges. Find out where your energy is going at work and determine who's in control: you or it?

"What is this life if, full of care We have no time to stand and stare."
W. H. DAVIES

Take a long, hard look at how you spend your time at work. Could you work more effectively so that you leave for home on time and not take anything with you?

Could you delegate more? If you were surer of your goals or what managers want, would that stop you wasting your time? Is there equipment you could get that would cut down any work that you're doing unnecessarily?

Take a leaf out of IDEA 39, *Give it a break*, and plan and take regular vacations. And don't forget to take the rest of the family!

Try another idea...

DELEGATE AT HOME IF YOU CAN

The daily plate-spinning act of work, school runs, childcare, and out-of-work activities goes on in most homes. Could you delegate more? You could employ a cleaner or a gardener, get some help with ironing or home decorating, link up with other parents to share the school run. Allocate jobs to your partner and the kids so that you're not doing more than your share—do what it takes, be it screaming, bribing, or begging.

Spend time negotiating roles between you and your partner. If you're caring for children or an elderly parent, take all the help you're offered or can afford. Don't be too proud to ask for or accept help from your friends and family—they want to help.

THINK OF YOUR FAMILY

Invest in the time you spend exclusively with your family. Put dedicated time aside at least once a week when your family does something together. This may be difficult, especially with teenagers who don't want to be seen out with their parents on pain of death by embarrassment, but do it anyway. It could be just sitting around the dinner table—at home or elsewhere—and discussing things that everyone is finding

"Enjoy yourself. It's later than you think."
CHINESE PROVERB

Defining idea...

stressful at work or school—a sort of gigantic debrief. Or you could all opt for a new activity that everyone can join, on equal terms—maybe a new sport, art, or craft. As you get interested in learning that new skill, sport, or hobby, it'll start to seem at least as important as your work, and help to rebalance your life.

How did it go?

Q   I always squeeze in time with my family, even when I'm really busy at work. How can I make them more appreciative of the effort I make?

A   *Time with your children and partner should be quality time, and not just times when you are too tired to do anything else. Try, try, and try again—to relax and give them your undivided attention when you are with them; don't let them think they are just filling your schedule until it's time for work again.*

Q   I prefer being at work to being on vacation and just count the days until I can check back in at work. Is that so wrong?

A   *Yes, you idiot! A vacation means just that. I bet you sneak your work into your carry-on luggage thinking that you'll catch up when the family or your partner is otherwise engaged. Leave your laptop and cell phone at home. You need to take a real break—you'll work more effectively when you return to work and all your coworkers will love you the more for it.*

27

Stress buster

Stress is like a virus. You're contagious if you have it and you pass it on to everyone around you. So, cool it and de-stress.

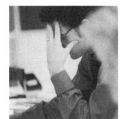

Don't tolerate stress. Change your environment as well as yourself. Pro-actively control stress-provoking factors at work. You may have to learn how to be more assertive. Don't let people put work on you.

STRESS AND BACK PAIN

Stress doesn't happen in a vacuum. Pressures and problems at home often overflow onto how someone feels and performs at work, and the effects of stress at work are often taken home and unfairly dumped there.

Stress is a very real problem that leads to a range of physical symptoms, including muscle tension and back pain. There may be psychological consequences, too, such as anxiety and depression, as well as increased risks of cancer and heart disease.

Here's an idea for you... Reduce the number or extent of your commitments. Cut down on unnecessary travel or out-of-work meetings. Redesign your garden so that it's easier to keep. If you don't have time to do something you're interested in, save it for later. Don't agree to stand as a candidate for your union, the neighborhood watch, or any other body, however flattered you are to be asked—unless you particularly want to and can give up something else to make time for it. Once you're running around less, you'll be more effective at work or have more quality time to relax or pursue your hobbies.

HOW YOU DEAL WITH PRESSURE

Stress can affect any one of us. But you may not realize that you're stressed. You may have been warned by others to "slow down" and have delighted in ignoring such advice and pushing yourself on regardless. How you deal with pressure is partly due to your personality and other life events that are going on around you. Solutions that work well for one person may not necessarily work as well, if at all, for someone else.

Become more aware of yourself and your reactions when you have symptoms of stress. Notice what provokes stress in you. Then you can consider what to do. Preventing things from getting too bad is the best form of stress management—the earlier you act, the better.

DEBRIEF

Talk things through. Even if it's not in your nature to confide in others, talk about your worries to those at work who are responsible for the stress you're under or are able to alleviate it. Seek the support of your colleagues, friends, and family. You'll feel better telling someone about your problems, and they may even have ideas to help reduce the sources of stress that are bugging you, or to help your back problems.

MANAGE YOUR TIME EFFICIENTLY

Time management is all about being smarter in getting through your work or chores at home. A certain degree of time pressure is probably necessary for you to maintain your interest and momentum in getting a job done. But too much pressure could tip you over the peak of your performance so that you're less efficient and your work or home life suffers.

Keep things in perspective and take a longer-term view rather than descend to short-term panic. See IDEA 29, *Say yes*, for more ideas about being positive and banishing negative thoughts and fears.

Try another idea...

THINK OF YOURSELF

You may feel that you can't let people down, whatever the costs to yourself. But there are limits, and if too much pressure is exerted on you for too long a time, you'll become burned out—and miserable from your back pain. So learn to control the demands on your time, before any excessive pressures affect you adversely.

Stress-proofing is what you need, so make time and space for yourself for fun, relaxation, hobbies, and enjoying simple pleasures. But do this as a way of life, not as an answer to a particular episode when you're already under par. Here's a good question for you—how much time have you spent in the last week on your own enjoyment?

"He who undertakes too much seldom succeeds."
DUTCH PROVERB

Defining idea...

123

Limit your workload so that you can enjoy an out-of-work life. Factor in enough time for having fun. Find methods of relaxation that work for you. Follow a healthy lifestyle—eating healthy foods, getting regular exercise, not smoking, limiting the amount of alcohol you drink. Look after your health. You need time for rest and recuperation like everyone else.

Learn to relax so that you can make the most of any free period, even a few minutes. Try and train yourself to shut right off from your surroundings. You'll need a quiet room with no disturbances at home, or even in your car.

PERSONAL SATISFACTION

Find time for personal and professional development—at work or with hobbies at home. To stay on top, you need to regain your enthusiasm for learning and your quest for knowledge and understanding. The personal satisfaction from completing a project, degree course, or other educational experience will make you feel more fulfilled and re-awaken your interest in life.

How did it go?

Q   **I sweat a lot. Does that mean I'm stressed?**

A   *Not necessarily—how many sweaters are you wearing? Seriously, we all experience stress in different ways. What one person feels is stressful may not be so for another person. If you're suffering from the bad effects of stress you might feel sweaty, have palpitations, have a dry mouth or headaches, lose your appetite for food, fun, or sex, eat too much or too little, lose interest in your appearance or in other people, be tearful, feel that everything is pointless. On the other hand, you might not be stressed at all—you might just sweat a lot.*

Q   **Trying to limit my workload means having to cut corners to get my work done and that causes me stress. What can I do?**

A   *Stop being a perfectionist. Accept that being "good enough" is good enough. Have you considered whether you're setting your personal standards too high and aiming for excellence too much of the time? Even if the pressure applied is by yourself, it can still be stressful.*

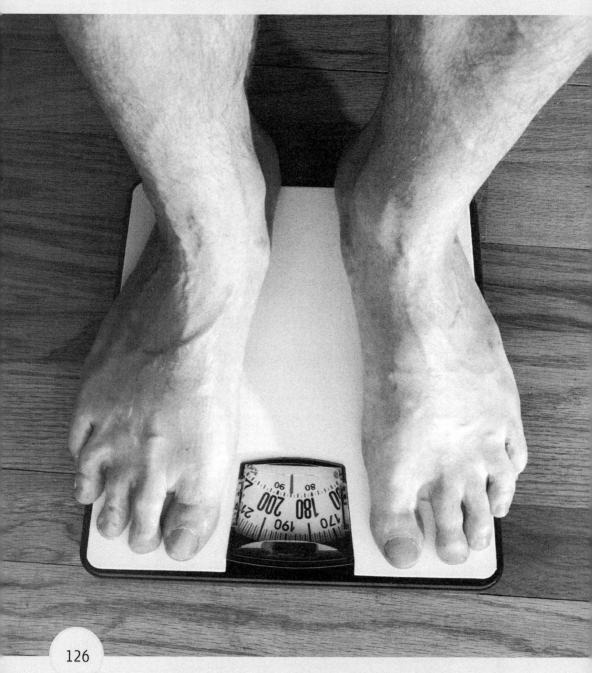

28

The big issue

You can't have too much of a good thing—except, perhaps, chocolate. Excess weight is like excess baggage—you'll pay for it eventually, unless you lose it.

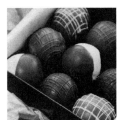

A big tummy strains your spine, spoiling its natural curves, making back pain more likely or more acute. It may be your excess blubber that's keeping your back pain going—so lose it, big man!

IT'S RISKY HAVING TOO BIG A BELLY

The worst place to carry excess fat is around your middle. Thinking about your general health rather than just your back problems, the relative distribution of fat between your waist and hips is a much better predictor of heart disease risk than your total weight to height ratio. Any man with a waist circumference that is more than 37 inches will have increased health risks from being overweight; the cut-off figure for a woman is 31.5 inches.

Here's an idea for you...

Find out how many calories you can burn off by everyday activities and what that looks like in terms of food. If you eat something extra it must be balanced with an equivalent extra energy output. For instance, driving a car for an hour will burn 80 calories (no matter the speed), which is equivalent to one slice of bread. Walking at 3 mph for an hour works off 260 calories, equivalent to 1.5 pints of beer or half a small pizza. Walking at 4 mph for an hour works off 420, while running at 5.5 mph works off 600. An hour of window cleaning or 30 minutes of gardening is equivalent to a large glass of wine or a small portion of ice cream, at 160 calories.

FOUR WAYS TO TACKLE YOUR EXCESS WEIGHT OR OBESITY

There are four approaches you can try to get rid of those extra pounds. If you've tried them all, think about your back problems and how bad the pain is, and try again.

First up, you could start by starting and maintaining a sensible diet. By sensible I really mean healthy—a diet in which the various food groups are well balanced.

Second, you could change your default feeding behavior. Stopping snacking between meals should automatically reduce your intake, even if it means you eat slightly more at mealtimes. Eating your main meals earlier in the day will help you avoid converting the spare calories to fat at night. Or join a weight-loss group to motivate you.

The third way is to start regular exercise or sports. If you can't stop shoveling the calories in, at least this way you'll burn them off.

Finally, there's drug treatment. This really is the last resort, and should only be used when all other approaches have been exhausted and for people who remain in the obese category.

For any of these approaches to work you must be motivated to change and determined to see them through over the medium to long term.

OKAY, YOU'VE HEARD THIS BEFORE, BUT LISTEN UP

Having trouble losing that weight? Usual diets not working? Why not check out IDEA 24, *Just a suggestion*, and see if hypnotherapy can crack it for you?

Try another idea...

Fat has over twice as many calories as starch or protein of the same weight. Beware of invisible fats, such as occur in foods like cookies, cakes, chocolate, pastry, and savory snacks. Read the labels. Trim fat from meat and poultry. Opt for lower fat milk, dairy products, and spreads. Choose to bake or grill rather than fry. Fill up on bread, cereals, potatoes, fruit, and vegetables. If you must snack, choose low-fat variants to suit your taste—everyone has their own favorites. It may be a little extreme to throw the food away and eat the packaging, but you get the idea.

BE REALISTIC ABOUT YOUR WEIGHT LOSS

Strict diets are difficult to sustain in the longer term. Some targets for you if you're really overweight or obese are 5.5 pounds weight loss in the first 4 weeks, or 5 percent of your body weight in the first three months. Go for a 10 percent reduction in your body weight by the end of one year. It's relatively easy to lose weight over a short period but much more difficult to maintain your weight loss over the longer term.

"The trouble with jogging is that the ice falls out of your glass."
MARTIN MULL, actor and satirist

Defining idea...

129

GET OUT OF THE BAR

Alcoholic drinks are full of hidden calories. A pint of beer is nearly 200 calories. A liter of wine is about 750 calories. So remember to include the calories that you're drinking, too, if you're on a calorie-counting diet.

How did it go?

Q I'm so hungry when I'm on a diet, I always give in and binge. What foods are best to fill up on when my stomach's growling?

A   *In general, foods with a high fiber content will fill you up and keep you full for longer. Learn to accept the feeling of hunger. Unfortunately, when you are on a diet you do tend to think of food more and feel hungry more often. But you don't need to eat just because you are hungry—that's a common mistake. And you certainly don't need to eat just because you are bored. Do some exercise instead.*

Q I'm bound to attend lots of business lunches. How can I resist the specialities of the house?

A   *Careful you don't let your guard slip when you're out with friends or on business. If you drink alcohol your resolve may crumble and you'll end up having that chocolate mousse or pudding after all. And boy, are some of those puddings loaded! Choose the low-fat options on the menu, whether or not they're your favorite foods. And keep to it—it'll be worth it in the end.*

29

Say yes

Heard of positive self-talk? If so, you've probably been talking to a shrink. Being positive makes sense. If you look on the positive side, you'll get the negative things in proportion—a tiny proportion.

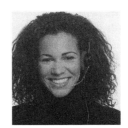

Concentrate on what you can do and not what you can't do.

WATCH YOUR WORDS

Stay positive about doing your everyday activities as per normal, despite your back pain. Play down your problem. Avoid using alarming words like "ruptured" if you're talking about your slipped disc. A "ruptured" disc conjures up the image of the disc being splattered on the inside of your spinal cord, which exaggerates your case (if it doesn't actually exaggerate your condition, try using the word "splattered"; nobody will take you seriously and it might rub off on you). Say "It hurts" rather than "I'm in agony." Minimize how it's affecting you.

ACCENTUATE THE POSITIVE

You may sometimes find yourself looking at things in a bleak manner, when your back pain seems never-ending. Constantly repeating negative thoughts to yourself

Here's an idea for you... **Draw a visual analog scale to try and quantify your pain and how restricted your movement is. Draw a horizontal line, and label it 0 at one end and 10 at the other—where 0 equals no pain and 10 equals unbearable pain, like you'd imagine childbirth could be without any pain relief. Then draw an X where you think the pain is on any one day. Draw a different colored X to mark how mobile you are. Put a date on your drawing and put it away in a drawer. Repeat the exercise once a week, and then every so often get all the records out to compare the gradings and chart your progress.**

will make you feel really frustrated about your pain and what it's stopping you from doing. Instead, make yourself use positive self-talk inside your head or to other people. Change negative words and statements to positive ones. Instead of saying "I'm worried about my back pain," say "I'm wondering about my back pain." Turn "I should" to "I could." Look at times when the negative event that you're dreading didn't happen when you were in a similar situation. Maybe your back pain didn't recur for several years once the previous episode was over. If you've got a straw, clutch at it.

ELIMINATE THE NEGATIVE

Challenge your negative beliefs. Look at different scenarios, and see yourself overcoming your negative beliefs step by step. For example, think about the variety of activities that your back pain is stopping you from doing. In reality, you can actually do some of them—maybe it'll take you a little longer to do, or maybe you'll have to modify the activity slightly, say, by going by car instead of walking—but you can do it.

Don't let other people regard you as disabled or you'll feel like an outsider. If others do tasks for you that you could do yourself with a little effort, you'll stop trying and may become more immobile. Do what you can and only ask for or accept help when you really need it.

Having said that, you need to accept the limitations determined by your back pain. So what if you can't clean your house from top to bottom or dig the garden over like you used to be able to do? Get things in perspective—there are lots of other things you can still do, and now you've got more time to spend doing them!

Don't get overwhelmed by demands—if things are piling up, find someone else to take on some of the jobs. Just prioritize and see what you can cope with. Don't feel guilty about circumstances outside your control—you know that you have to limit what you can do until your back improves. Make positive plans for when you are better.

Be practical. Search through catalogs for equipment you can buy to get tasks or chores done without straining your back.

For other tips on how to live with your limitations, see IDEA 50, *Living as a different you*.

Try another idea...

SMILE

Think positive thoughts. Look for the humor in a situation whenever you can and enjoy life, despite your back pain. Use positive body language, rather than gloomy inactivity.

"Once you replace negative thoughts with positive ones, you'll start having positive results."
WILLIE NELSON

Defining idea...

MEASURE YOUR PROGRESS

Sometimes pain seems to go on and on and on. But if you bother to look back and remember exactly how bad you were at the outset, you'll realize that you are in fact getting better slowly. It's difficult to measure the exact extent of the back pain you're experiencing.

133

Q **I'm miserable because I can't play squash anymore. What else can I do?**

A *Find a new hobby or activity to do. If you're not able to do a favorite hobby any more because of your back problems, then replace it with one you can do. You could grow to enjoy it just as much. If swinging a sports club or racket is impossible, then take up walking or cycling. If climbing mountains is beyond you now, could sailing give you the same thrill with less strain on your back? If gymnastics or archery is out, would dancing or bowling keep your back more supple?*

Q **I don't seem to have as many friends as I used to since I stopped playing sports because of my back pain, and now I'm bored. Should I just be patient?**

A *It sounds to me as if you are giving up—and that's an absolute no-no. Take up new hobbies that you're able to do and you'll soon get a new circle of friends. Don't let the subject of your back pain dominate your conversation with other people. If they ask, okay then you can tell them, but quickly move on to another topic of conversation. No one likes a whiner who goes on about their health problems all the time; they'd rather talk about their own.*

30

Back to work

Fail to prepare? Then prepare to fail. If work caused your back pain in the first place, or if work makes it worse, then plan smart ways around the likely problems—but don't loaf around at home.

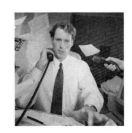

Most back pain gets better by itself. And it's helped if you get back to work and undertake your normal activities as soon as possible, despite your back pain.

ADAPT YOUR JOB

When you first go back to work, you may have to reorganize what you do so there's less strain on your back until you're fully recovered. If you normally do heavy lifting, you'll be able to return to work sooner if your employer can find you a lighter job for a while.

Look at your working environment to see if there's anything you can change about the way you work. Look at the ergonomics there. Think about how you lift weighty objects, whether they are a core part of your work or an incidental activity as part of working in an office. Maybe you could use a hoist or trolley to make the lifting easier for you.

Here's an
idea for
you...

Try to boost your job satisfaction. If you're satisfied and interested in your job, that will stress-proof you against those parts that you find stressful. Decide what success at work looks like for you and stick with that as far as possible. Is it money, power, making people better? Talk to a trusted colleague to decide if your goals are realistic. Now work out your tactics. Plan for several quick wins in the next few months and at least one longer term goal to invest time and effort in.

KEEP WORK IN PERSPECTIVE

Just because you're back at work doesn't mean that you should go straight back to your bad old ways. If you return to a high-pressure job where you flog yourself to work all hours, you'll be out sick again pretty soon. So keep work in perspective and overcome the seven deadly sins of the workaholic, as follows:

1   Stop being a perfectionist.
2   Don't judge your mistakes too harshly.
3   Resist the desire to control everything.
4   Learn to assertively decline extra commitments if you are already pressed for time.
5   Look after your personal health and fitness.
6   Allow time for personal growth, the family, and leisure.
7   Don't be too proud to ask for help.

BEING HAPPY AT WORK

Find ways to be happy at work, so that you go home relaxed and satisfied, not frazzled and resentful. Take time to think about your job and review the high points. Keep off the treadmill where all you can think about is having too little time to do your job properly, if at all. Beware of the activity trap—resist becoming addicted to

Defining
idea...

"Find a job you like and you add five days to every week."
H. JACKSON BROWN JR, writer

constant activity and the adrenaline buzz that gives you. Don't confuse success with endless activity.

Don't be anxious—be happy. If you feel anxious, explore the reasons why. Don't work to other people's agendas all the time, chasing unrealistic targets. If you think their targets are unachievable, discuss what other resources can be made available to enable you to hit them. Try to tackle the causes of your anxiety. Bring back the fun and satisfaction in your working life.

Don't burn out, and don't forget to switch off from work when you leave for home. Pace yourself and create your preventive health plan for a balanced life, as in IDEA 26, *Get a life.*

Try another idea...

Prioritize tasks and responsibilities at work in order of their importance rather than their urgency. Find better and smarter ways to do things more easily, and don't battle with an overload of work. Avoid "hurry-sickness."

CUT DOWN ON STRESS AT WORK

Work may be a cause of stress for you. Or it may be that your general symptoms of stress are obvious at work. Whatever, stress will make it difficult for you to concentrate and your performance at work may well fall under par. You'll spend your time wishing you could avoid work. If you're stressed, you'll feel tired at work and may take time off sick. So identify what's causing that stress, and try to minimize it. Talk to colleagues and see if they feel the same, and seek their support to draw up an action plan.

"The human race is faced with a cruel choice: work or daytime television."
ANONYMOUS

Defining idea...

How did
it go?

Q   I'm wondering about a different career. My work is making my back ache through all the lifting I'm forced to do and the stress I'm under. What should I do?

A   *Sounds as if you need help to figure out your career plans. To make a rational career choice you first need to know a good deal about yourself—your strengths and weaknesses, your personal preferences and dislikes—and then find out the type of work that is a good fit with your personality and nature. You could consult a career counselor now—they can help at any stage of your working life. It's never too late.*

Q   I have to travel long distances at work and all that driving is crippling me. Any ideas on how I can cope?

A   *If you normally drive long distances to meetings, maybe you can hold them by video conferencing or using a webcam by your desk. Alternatively, you could organize your sales through telephone group discussions. Maybe the people you usually go to see would be willing to travel to you for a change—a day out of the office and all that. Perhaps you could still do the traveling but use the train or plane instead of your car. That way, you can move around more during the journey to ease your back. If all these are impractical, try changing your car to one with better seats.*

31

"Not tonight, darling— I have a backache"

Foreplanning is just as important as foreplay for finding positions that suit you both.

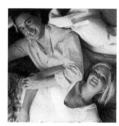

Good sex stretches your back and spontaneously loosens the joints of your spine. Who says you can't have your cake and eat it, too?

FIND A POSITION TO SUIT YOU

If your back's painful you'll probably opt for conventional positions on the bed— having sex in a closet or in the car, with the sort of contortions they require, might well upset your back even if you weren't in pain before you started. And that pain will be a turn off, and your sexual feelings will just wither away. So be aware of your body and don't get into awkward positions likely to trigger your jigger.

PREPARE WELL

Get yourself as comfortable as possible. Try taking a painkiller an hour or so before you expect to have sex, so that it has a chance to work and dull any pain. Undress carefully first. You don't want to be struggling to get your clothes off in a cramped

Ask your partner to massage your back as a preliminary to sex. Using oils will make the massage smoother. Get them to knead your back muscles. Experiment with a back roller or vibrating tool, as well as or instead of their hands. See what it takes to soothe and relax you. If your back's up to it, return the favor and massage their back, too, but be careful not to twist.

position and have your back lock. Alternatively, buy a seductive dressing gown that you can change into and slip off easily.

Settle onto your bed or other firm surface. Don't rush, take your time, and enjoy yourself. Let your partner know how they can help you. As good sex is about pleasing your partner, they shouldn't mind making it right for you. But don't let them treat you like an invalid and be frightened of hurting you, or having sex will become a medical event rather than the good time both of you want and expect.

PLAY DOCTORS 'N' NURSES?

Well you could play at being the patient and let your partner be the doctor or nurse. They could examine your back, massage it and lovingly caress it, turn you over and...you can imagine the rest. If you like that, the next step could be for one or both of you to dress up for the role!

Make a play for their sympathy. Use the medical jargon you pick up from your medical notes or the Internet. Don't just say I've got a "sore shoulder," say I've got a "suprascapular bursitis"—that must be worth a loving massage.

Work to make sex fun. The more you're distracted from your back pain, the better. Perhaps you can tell each other stories or jokes. You could role-play celebrities. The more fun it is, the more you'll forget about your back problems.

WHEN SOMEBODY LOVES YOU BACK

Try to ignore your back problem and find a way to have a regular sex life, experimenting with different positions and supports. Otherwise you'll get frustrated and may become depressed and solitary. You need to lead as normal a life as possible with your partner. Sex should distract you from your back problems. The more you focus on your pain to the exclusion of everything else, the more your pain will dominate your life. Sex will raise your spirits and put you in a cheerier mood.

If your back is painful or stiff, lie on a heating pad for a while first so your back muscles are more relaxed. See IDEA 10, *Some like it hot*, to read more about heat treatments.

Try another idea...

LET ME TOUCH YOU FOR A WHILE

Try to inject some freshness into your relationship with your partner, to strengthen your bond. Make a date, just like you did in the old days, and try to arrange regular outings around shared interests. Acknowledge any problems with your sex life if they exist. These are usually due to communication difficulties or lack of time alone together. If you make rebuilding your relationship a priority, you'll probably find some fun and laughter bubbling to the surface.

Keep working at establishing good and continuing communication in a marriage or long-term relationship. Consider visiting a counselor together if your relationship is under threat. And see them sooner rather than later, or it could be too late.

"The most intolerable pain is produced by prolonging the keenest pleasure."
GEORGE BERNARD SHAW

Defining idea...

141

How did it go? **Q I dread my back hurting when we have sex, and it's preventing me from getting into the right mood. What should we do?**

A *You're right that the responsibility to get into the mood is up to both of you, not you alone. Try heat on your back—get that rug out in front of your fire. Put on music that relaxes you both. Alcohol might help to put you in the mood and relax you, too—but don't imbibe so much that it dulls your feelings and makes it difficult to have sex at all.*

Q What sexual positions can I try, as my back is bad at the moment?

A *So long as your partner is aware of your back problem, you should be able to find a position to suit you both. Talk about it before you get into foreplay. Maybe a side-to-side position will suit you best, rather than lying on your back with your partner's weight on top, or being on top of your partner when your back will be unsupported. There are lots of positions to choose from so you should find some ways of lying together that are pain-free. Buy the* Kama Sutra *if you need any more ideas—or dig out the secret one you bought as a youngster and that your mom used to borrow without your knowledge.*

32

Hurt so bad

Whoever said "just say no" to drugs clearly never had to live with chronic back pain. When you're in crippling pain and it's putting a stopper on your lifestyle, say yes to painkillers.

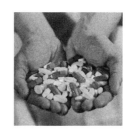

Backache ruining your life? Pain killing your enjoyment? Then do a little pain-killing yourself courtesy of the pharmacist.

WHAT DRUGS ARE OUT THERE?

Not all painkillers are the same, so it's important to know what's out there, and what they'll do for you and to you.

Acetaminophen sounds boring—everyone has some somewhere in the house—but it really is one of the best types of medication for back pain. If it doesn't work for you, it could be because your back pain is just too severe. On the other hand, you might not be taking enough, or expecting it to cure rather than relieve your pain. So try taking eight 500-milligram tablets spread out over 24 hours, unless you're taking other prescribed medication that would clash with acetaminophen or already contains it. Side effects of acetaminophen are rare, and pain relief lasts for 4–6 hours. Stock up with acetaminophen from the supermarket or your pharmacist.

Here's an idea for you...

Want some pain relief but not happy about popping pills? Then try painkillers in cream form. There is a wide range of anti-inflammatory creams on the market. Capsaicin cream is used to treat chronic pain and could be just the thing for your back problem. Ask your pharmacist.

Another drug you can buy easily is ibuprofen, which is classed as a non-steroidal anti-inflammatory drug. Taken at regular intervals (e.g., 200 milligrams 3 times a day), ibuprofen will relieve straightforward backache. Drugs like ibuprofen can cause stomach problems, such as indigestion, nausea, diarrhea, and even bleeding from a stomach ulcer, though the latter is uncommon. They may make problems with blood pressure or asthma worse in susceptible people. Ibuprofen is more effective than acetaminophen for relieving back pain as it acts on the inflammation causing the problem as well as relieving the pain. It may be cheaper to get a prescription for a bigger quantity of ibuprofen if you need a high dose (e.g., 600 milligrams 3 times a day) or take it over a long time. Take it with food to lessen the chances of getting any side effects.

If acetaminophen is not strong enough to tackle your pain, your doctor might prescribe you stronger painkillers, like codydramol or co-codamol. More powerful still are drugs like dihydrocodeine, which are long-distant relatives of opium. These opiate drugs have side effects such as constipation, and may even depress your breathing rate and cause drowsiness, confusion, nausea and vomiting, or an itchy allergic rash.

Defining idea...

"I never read a patent medicine advertisement without being impelled to the conclusion that I am suffering from a particular disease therein dealt with."
JEROME K. JEROME

Another tack is to try a muscle relaxant. If your back pain has arisen from muscle spasm, or you've got spasm as your body's reaction to your back pain, you might be prescribed a muscle relaxant such as baclofen or diazepam.

They can be effective in reducing your acute back pain, but they do have drowsiness as a side effect. You also may develop dependency, even after courses as short as a week.

So you don't want to take painkillers, but doing nothing is not an option either? Look at IDEA 17, *It's electric*, for how a TENS machine could help you.

Try another idea…

Antidepressants are prescribed for chronic lower back pain, just as for other types of long-standing pain. Having pain over a long time can actually make you depressed, but antidepressant drugs are used to relieve pain when other treatments have failed, even in people who are not depressed. Amitriptyline is used for pain relief at lower doses than those used in depression, e.g., 10–50 milligrams a day, but may still give you side effects such as a dry mouth, sleepiness, and constipation.

Anticonvulsant drugs that are usually used for epilepsy can be prescribed by a doctor in similar doses to relieve pain. Antidepressants will be tried first as they may cause fewer side effects than anticonvulsants.

If your local doctor can't relieve your pain sufficiently, they might send you to a pain clinic.

Another option instead of your doctor's pills is to buy glucosamine, which is available over the counter in a pharmacy or health food shop and is classed as a complementary medicine. It can be taken as a pill or as an injection into a muscle. It's used for arthritis, so if this is the cause of your back problems, it might be worth trying.

"Half of the modern drugs could well be thrown out of the window, except the birds might eat them."
DR. MARTIN HENRY FISCHER

Defining idea…

How did it go?

Q   **I do take acetaminophen, but the pain keeps coming back just as bad as ever. Should it do this?**

A   *It's better to take painkillers at regular intervals to control pain rather than take as necessary. Don't wait for the pain to return—zap it before it gets back on its feet. Take acetaminophen four times a day until the pain has subsided.*

Q   **Should I take painkillers at all? Won't masking the pain mean that I could damage my numbed back without realizing it by movements that put it under more strain?**

A   *If taking painkillers means that you can stay active, then that is good for your back in general, and an active life is much more enjoyable. Painkillers are not wonder drugs—you'll still be able to feel some pain through them to warn you if you put your back in an awkward position. A word of warning, though: You must also avoid overusing painkillers. Taking painkillers several times per week over a considerable time may cause rather than relieve headaches, especially those containing caffeine or codeine. A good rule of thumb is not to use painkillers for more than 7 days a month if possible.*

33

At the cutting edge

Occasionally, a symptom might flag a condition you will really wish you didn't have. Doc, what can you do to help?

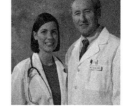

There are some well-recognized "red flags" that indicate you might have a serious condition. So take note if your symptoms are flagged here.

GETTING MEDICAL HELP

Self-help's all well and good, but if your back pain's not getting better, it's worth consulting your family doctor or therapist. They'll want to know when your back pain started, the site of the pain, if it radiates down your legs, your occupation, any previous problems, any medication you're on, what your general health is like, about your lifestyle or any recent injury. All these are clues to the cause of your back pain for these health sleuths.

They'll examine how your spine moves, extend your legs straight relative to your spine, watch you walk, tap your reflexes, and observe how tender your spine is. They may examine other parts of your body, too, if they think your back pain is part of a bigger picture. Then there'll be discussion about whether you need urgent investigation or simple treatment.

Here's an idea for you... If you need surgery, find out about less invasive options, such as microscopic surgery, rather than full-blown surgery to take out an intervertebral disc. Coblation nucleoplasty is a new treatment for partly slipped discs done as an outpatient procedure. It uses a radio-frequency probe to vaporize the part of the disc causing the pressure effects. Another treatment for compression fractures of the vertebrae resulting from osteoporosis is a kind of bone cement to fix the fractured bone.

SERIOUS CAUSES OF BACK PAIN

Lower back pain has many causes. By now you know about the most likely diagnoses of simple backache or slipped disc. Some serious causes of backache include infection, tumor, osteoporosis, rheumatoid arthritis, fracture, or inflammation. One in every 100 people consulting their family doctor with back pain will have cancer, 4 percent will have a compression fracture, and up to 3 percent a slipped intervertebral disc. A really unusual source of back pain is an aneurysm of the aortic artery that travels up the center of your body, at the level of your abdomen, when it's about to rupture.

IT'S A RED FLAG DAY

You should see a doctor right away if your back pain is getting worse for no apparent reason. Red flags are: a significant injury, such as from a road accident or fall from a height; having cancer elsewhere in your body; presenting with severe back pain for the first time under age 20 or over 55 years old; being generally unwell or losing weight; being on steroid drugs or abusing drugs; or progressively worsening pain not related to movement. Other serious symptoms or signs are difficulty in urinating or opening your bowels, or developing pain in your thoracic spine (the part at chest level). The docs will worry if they note widespread signs and symptoms showing that the nerves in your body are not functioning right, or that you have a structural deformity of your spine.

If your family doctor or therapist spot any of these red flags, they'll order X-rays or other investigations and may refer you to a specialist as an emergency, depending on how urgent your problem is.

WHEN YOU SHOULD SEE A SPECIALIST

Find out as much information as possible using the sources described in IDEA 52, *Nothing is beyond your reach*, so you can have an intelligent conversation about the risks and benefits of an operation with the surgeon.

Try another idea...

See a specialist as an emergency or urgent case if you have difficulty controlling your bladder or bowels, progressive weakness of your muscles, numbness around your back passage and genital areas, or numbness, pins and needles, or weakness in both legs. These indicate that nerve roots are trapped on both sides of your body. This is the cauda equina syndrome. It might be that you have a centrally slipped disc, abscess, or tumor pressing on nerves running from your lower spine to supply feeling and power to your anal and genital areas. The specialist will do imaging investigations, and operate to relieve pressure on nerves that are compressed so much that you cannot urinate or defecate.

Surgery should only be considered where simpler treatments have failed. It's really for treating nerve root problems that are not getting better or for the cauda equina

"The doctor is to be feared more than the disease."
LATIN PROVERB

Defining idea...

syndrome. Surgery involves the removal of the already slipped disc along with any loose parts of the disc, worn bone, or facet joint structures near the nerve root. Occasionally, when the spine seems unstable and other treatments have failed, two or more vertebrae may be fused using bone grafts.

Q **I've had a really bad bout of sciatica going down my left leg for three weeks and it's just not getting any better. My family doctor keeps reassuring me, but should I insist on seeing a specialist?**

A *Whoa—wait a bit. Give it time. Your family doctor will want you to see a specialist if you have a pinched nerve that's not getting better after 6 weeks. The specialist may then investigate further, or try different treatments like a steroid or trigger point injection, or organize manual or electrical therapies. If it's just simple back pain that you've got that hasn't improved and is preventing you from resuming your normal activities, say, 3 months later, your doctor may refer you to a specialist then.*

Q **I'm still relatively young, in my mid-forties. Are the risks from spinal surgery worth taking?**

A *You're right, there are risks with surgery. You can react to the anesthetic, or develop a blood clot that might lodge in your leg, lungs, heart, or brain. You can hemorrhage so badly that you require a blood transfusion. Or damage could be done to your spinal cord, with a remote risk of you being paralyzed for life. Even with the best surgeon, you're at risk. So only go for back surgery as a last resort. But it's your call.*

34

Moving forward

Don't beat yourself up about what you can't do. Focus on what you can do, then get out there and do it. Mind over matter puts you in control.

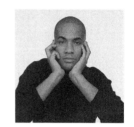

Don't let pain dominate your whole life and make you feel depressed and apathetic.

If you have a passive attitude to your health and back problems then you're more likely to develop chronic back pain. Your psychological state can affect how quickly you get better and whether your back pain comes back. There are a variety of "yellow flags" that indicate someone with negative attitudes, beliefs, and behaviors in relation to their back pain. If this is you, shake them off, or your back pain may stay as a feature of your life. The more of these flags that apply to you, the worse your outlook. But remember—with a positive attitude you can do something about most, if not all, of them.

BEAT THOSE YELLOW FLAGS

You may feel that you've lost control of your life and cease to struggle to overcome the pain. Back pain may keep you awake at night so that being chronically tired compounds your low mood and general negative perspective of life. If you see your back pain as harmful or potentially severely disabling, start thinking positively.

Here's an idea for you... **Get motivated. Buy an exercise video that covers back and joint activities and join in. It'll take you through a whole routine of balanced exercises that you can repeat every day, and help maintain your motivation. Invite a friend to do it with you to make it more fun.**

Don't avoid moving because you fear that you'll trigger your back pain—grit your teeth and go for it. Just because you've been out of work with back pain before doesn't mean you can't work now because of it. If you're generally in a low mood and have lost interest in things, do something about it—get your social life back, for a start.

If you're obviously stressed—anxious, angry, frustrated, or have difficulty concentrating, difficulty sleeping, poor appetite, lost your sex drive, and are depressed—seek help from a doc or talk things through with a friend.

EXPECT IT TO GET BETTER

Believe that your back pain is not serious. With time, it will get better, especially if you try some of the brilliant ideas here. Keep repeating to yourself that light physical activity is not harmful, and is the way for you to get better. Read more about getting better with various treatments. Feel reassured. There are lots of educational leaflets and booklets that'll help you manage your back pain yourself. They should help you to trust the advice to stay active.

Defining idea... *"A strong positive mental attitude will create more miracles than any wonder drug."*
PATRICIA NEAL, actor

PRACTICE RELAXATION

The benefits of relaxation lie in making you feel better as well as the actual physical relaxation of your muscles and the concomitant relief of pain.

WORK AND GETTING FIT

Stay at work, or return to work as soon as you can. As well as the activity being beneficial, being with your colleagues should raise your spirits—it's easy to get gloomy about your back pain if you're by yourself at home most of the time. And you need to keep a regular paycheck coming in. Take the painkillers offered so that you can tolerate your back pain and go about your business as normal.

Getting in shape and improving your general health will have lots of positive benefits on your general well-being in addition to your specific back problem.

Some complementary therapies that are used for back pain also have good effects on the mind. Look up IDEA 14, *Strike a pose*, or IDEA 25, *Let's put you in the picture*.

Try another idea...

PHONE A FRIEND

Talk to other people who manage to live with their back problems without letting it get them down. Let them put your back pain into perspective and let their positive outlook infect you. Maybe seeing a counselor would help, especially if you have other problems with, say, your relationships or financial matters. If you restore your marriage or make a decision about separation, you may be able to move on and put the problem of your back pain behind you. A financial adviser could help you sort matters out if that's an issue, and your back pain will then seem of less importance.

"If you can believe it, the mind can achieve it."
RONNIE LOTT, football player

Defining idea...

How did
it go? **Q** **I've been out of work because of my back pain for ages. I just sit
around and watch TV and feel sorry for myself. How do I get
myself motivated?**

A *Congratulations! You're partway there already, as asking about it shows
you're contemplating making a change to your lifestyle. The next stage is to
plan the change and then...do it! So plan to increase the amount of
physical activity you take. Try to find a buddy to do it with, so you can spur
each other on when one of you can't be bothered. Join a gym and if your
resolve to visit it ever wavers, just remind yourself how much the
membership cost! Do a few minutes' exercise every day and build up from
there.*

Q **I'm depressed because my back pain just isn't getting better. What
can I do?**

A *A course of antidepressant drugs from your family doctor might help to
reverse your depression, and they can help with your pain control, too.
You'll need to be on them for at least six months to get their full effect. A
counselor is another alternative—they may help you to see that you're using
your back pain as a way of avoiding normal life and give you more insight
into how to overcome your health problems.*

35

Relief on the inside, life on the outside

Do doctors give you the needle? You'll hope so if your symptoms get better with a pain-relieving injection. What a site for sore thighs if you have sciatica.

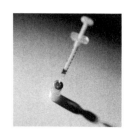

A shot could relieve your pain and allow you freer movement.

Various drugs can give you relief for your back pain if injected over the painful area of your spine. An injection is sometimes used to help make a diagnosis as well as to treat severe pain that's not getting better.

EPIDURAL INJECTIONS

One main reason for having an epidural injection is chronic sciatica. If the source of your pain is from a slipped disc that is pressing on a nerve root, then the injection will be given into the epidural space between the spinal sac and the inside of the spinal canal. This enables the drugs injected to flow up and down the spine to coat the nerve roots near to the injection sites. The injection will be done under either local or general anesthetic.

The injection is a mix of local anesthetic and steroid. This relieves your pain through its anti-inflammatory action and frees adhesions around the nerve roots.

Here's an idea for you... **Ask the doctor or therapist treating you about having a spinal injection if your back pain's not getting better despite exercise or electrical or manual therapies. If they don't give spinal injections or can't explain why an injection shouldn't be tried, ask for a second opinion. Tell them you want to have a stab at one.**

The steroid part of the injection acts on the local area into which it's injected, reducing swelling and thus easing the compression of the nerve root. The effects of the local anesthetic wear off after a few hours, but if it relieves your pain for that time, the doctor or therapist will know she's hit the right spot. Sometimes a strong painkiller like morphine or fentanyl might be added to the mix, to give you more pain relief.

The steroid or cortisone that is injected is insoluble, so it stays around where it's injected. It's slowly broken down there, rather than being transported into the bloodstream and around the body. This means you'll avoid the generalized side effects that you'd have if you'd taken the steroid treatment orally. You won't notice any benefit right away, and it might be painful for the first day or two until the steroid starts working, but when it does, its effects can last for months. Epidural injections are relatively safe. Some patients complain of headaches or nausea afterward, but then some patients will complain about anything.

INJECTING TRIGGER POINTS

A doctor or an expert therapist might inject a mixture of steroid and local anesthetic into a trigger point of a painful ligament. Trigger points are small areas of muscle that have become tense over the years. The chronic muscle tension might have come about from poor posture, or anxiety and anger bottled up over the years. The pain from these trigger points radiates out elsewhere, so pain from, say, your lower back might radiate to one of your buttocks. Sometimes you are unaware of the trigger points until your back is massaged, then—ouch!

INJECTING FACET JOINTS

The facet joints are the joints that connect the vertebrae and protect the spinal cord. They tend to deteriorate with age. You can find out if your facet joints are painful by arching backward while you are standing up, as this movement puts pressure on them.

Go to a medical library or look on the Internet to find out more about what you'd be letting yourself in for with a spinal injection. Read about the risks and contraindications on the websites given in IDEA 52, *Nothing is beyond your reach.*

Try another idea...

The procedure for injection differs between centers. You'll probably have been investigated by a magnetic resonance imaging scan before having the injection. You might be partly sedated with a drug like valium, given as a pill some time before the procedure is done. Fluroscopy can be used to ensure that the needle's in the right position before the drug's injected. A magnified X-ray of your bony area will be projected as a TV image, so that the practitioner can see what she's doing. Sometimes a second or third injection will be given a week or more later if the first one proves ineffective.

SACRO-ILIAC JOINT INJECTIONS

As before, injecting a mix of a local anesthetic with a steroid helps to confirm the sacro-iliac joint as the real site of the pain, rather than the pain you're feeling radiating there from elsewhere. Again, the precise location is pinpointed by fluroscopy or other types of X-rays—and then, pow!

"Pain is inevitable. Suffering is optional."
ANONYMOUS

Defining idea...

How did **Q   I'm having an epidural injection tomorrow, and to be honest I have**
it go?   **no idea what it is. Can you tell me more about the actual**
                 procedure?

A   *Certainly. You'll be advised not to eat or drink for at least 6 hours before
your injection, in case you vomit. The injection will be done under sterile
conditions. The site might be numbed with a preliminary injection of local
anesthetic. If the epidural injection is going into your lumbar spine, the
needle will be inserted between two vertebrae. The practitioner will
cautiously monitor the effects of injecting a little of the drug first, and
then, when certain that the needle's in the right position, give you the full
dose.*

Q   Is there any reason why I shouldn't have a spinal injection?

A   *You won't be able to have a spinal injection if you're taking blood-thinning
warfarin, and you may be asked to stop taking aspirin or ibuprofen for a few
days before. If you have a local or general infection, then a spinal injection
might encourage its spread to your brain through the spinal canal. So tell
your practitioner about any wounds or rashes you've got anywhere.
Obviously you couldn't have a spinal injection if you were known to be
allergic to any of the drugs used. They are also not advisable if there is
nothing wrong with you.*

36

Why not have an X-ray?

Look at X-rays as you would a hungry Rottweiler. That's right—be frightened. Run away as fast as you can. X-rays are dangerous and rarely required.

Even under intense interrogation, X-rays don't give away much information. And they're crafty—they can look normal even when something's up and so lull you into a false sense of security.

NO X-RAYS, PLEASE

Simple back pain, like muscle strain, ligament, or facet joint strain, doesn't normally require X-rays. The soft moving tissues of your spine are all radiotranslucent, so any problem with your ligaments, muscles, tendons, nerve roots, and discs that causes pain will not show up on an X-ray. Your bones might show up well, and hey, it's nice to know they're still there, but so what? In fact, people can have serious conditions affecting their bones but still look normal on an X-ray, because it takes time for diseases such as cancer or infection to destroy the bone sufficiently for it to show up.

Routine X-rays are not recommended for investigating lower back pain lasting less than six weeks unless there are unusual signs to alert the doctor or therapist to the

Here's an idea for you...

Don't try to bully your doctor or therapist to arrange an X-ray on your back. Listen to their advice, and if they don't expect an X-ray to give them any new information, leave it at that. There's no point being exposed to X-rays for no possible benefit. If you do manage to get that X-ray done and it comes back normal, what will that tell you? That your back is normal or there's something wrong that doesn't show up on the X-ray. Happy now?

possibility you have a serious disease. A back X-ray is called for if you've been in an accident, or are generally unwell and your back pain is just one of many serious-sounding symptoms. If the pain persists for many weeks, or you've got nerve root compression, continuing inflammation, or other sinister symptoms, then you'll probably be X-rayed. However, as X-rays of the thoracic, lumbar, or sacral spine may not show a fracture, tumor, infection, or osteoporosis, a normal X-ray can be falsely reassuring. And even if the medics do spot something on your X-ray, they might not be able to tell if it's benign or malignant. Your doctor is likely to need more sophisticated imaging tests to discern the cause if you have worrying symptoms or signs, or if your back pain doesn't improve.

There's no need for your back to be X-rayed before a therapist undertakes manipulation.

MAGNETIC RESONANCE IMAGING (MRI) SCANNING

An MRI scan uses a large magnet instead of X-rays to get a picture of your spine. There's no need to have one of these scans if you only have simple lower back pain; this highly specialized (and therefore expensive) test is only justified when there are clinical indications of a problem with your spine. This is when symptoms persist or are severe, and could be indicative of an intervertebral disc problem that doctors think might require surgery or some other serious cause for your back pain. Not all abnormalities seen on a scan mean anything important. The scan picks up all sorts of tiny changes in your spine, many of which are due to you getting older. The MRI scan is just part of the evidence, not the whole story.

Remember that tests and treatments for back pain can be harmful although they're meant to help, as IDEA 48, *Trick or treat?*, will remind you.

Try another idea...

You will undergo an MRI scan as an outpatient. You lie on a special bed in a cylindrical machine that contains a powerful electromagnet. It's a tightly enclosed area and you must stay very still for however long it takes, which could be up to half an hour. An MRI scan is generally preferred to computed tomography as it gives a wider field of view and avoids the use of X-rays. The radiowaves that scan you produce high-quality images of the part of your body being focused upon, in cross section. It's the investigation of choice for evaluating mechanical disorders of the spine and any possible spinal infections.

ISOTOPE BONE SCANS

Bone scans can be useful when a spinal tumor is suspected from the medical history or physical examination. The scan might give more information or corroborate blood tests or X-ray findings. The whole skeleton can be visualized by the scan.

DISCOGRAPHY

Discography is useful if you can't have an MRI scan or if the MRI scan has not given enough information. It gives a 3-D reconstruction of your spine. A special fluid is injected into the nucleus of a disc to act as a contrast medium to show up the structure when viewed under X-ray. If the disc is healthy the contrast medium stays in the center of the spine. If the disc has prolapsed, the contrast medium will spread through the extent of the prolapse.

How did it go?

Q   The doctors have been telling me for years that my back pain is due to arthritis, but a recent back X-ray didn't show any sign of this. How can I trust what the doctors have said, what can my pain be due to, and why are they lying to me?

A   *Whoa, check the paranoia! X-rays are not a good guide as to how severe arthritis is. Plenty of people whose spine X-rays show wear and tear changes have few or no symptoms, just as there are people with a great deal of back pain who are believed to have osteoarthritis but have normal-looking X-rays. Don't lose faith in your doctor just because of one inconclusive result.*

Q   I think you're being alarmist. How can a quick photo of my spine by X-ray be dangerous, really?

A   *Three standard X-ray views of the lumbar spine involve 120–150 times the radiation dose of a chest X-ray. If you're very unlucky, you could die from exposure to radiation from X-rays of your spine. Is that alarmist enough for you?*

37

Things aren't what they used to be

It's that age-old problem—your bones thin as you get older. Just like money, osteoporosis runs in families, but it's not as easy to lose.

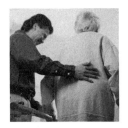

Unfortunately you can't swap your parents, but you can stay fit and active and eat a diet rich in calcium.

DEM BONES, DEM BONES

Osteoporosis is thinning of the bones. It's a degenerative bone disease that occurs over your lifetime. Therefore osteoporosis usually manifests in elderly people, though younger people who take steroid or thyroid drugs can suffer from it, too. Women who have an early menopause are more likely to get osteoporosis. It runs in families.

The low bone mass and low mineral density that are characteristic of osteoporosis mean your bones are more brittle and more prone to fracture. One in five women gets a vertebral fracture in her lifetime. Many women don't know it because they either have no real symptoms or don't see anyone about their pain—they just put up with it.

Here's an idea for you... **You can prevent osteoporosis to some extent–so don't be bone idle. People who do too little activity will get thinner bones. So do regular weight-bearing exercise. The best type of physical activity is one that physically stresses the bone, such as jumping, running, and skipping. Try twice-weekly exercise classes. That will increase bone density in adolescents, maintain it in young adults, and slow its decline in older age. If teenagers build up their bone density, they'll be less likely to get a fracture in later life.**

Everyone's bone density decreases as they get older. In young people the bones are really strong and are only crushed in severe injuries, such as from a road traffic accident. In men the bone density decreases by about 0.3 percent per year after their mid- to late twenties, while in women it declines by 0.5 percent per year, and sometimes as much as 2–3 percent per year after menopause. One in three women and one in twelve men over 50 years old have some degree of osteoporosis. Women who have late onset of periods coupled with early menopause have a greatly increased risk of developing osteoporosis.

There are some diseases with which osteoporosis is associated. Some, like thyrotoxicosis, are treatable; others, like cancer and some rheumatic disorders, can be more difficult to control.

WHY PAIN?

Pain comes about when bones partly or fully collapse. Additional pain arises from the curve or change in the structure of your spine, which compresses the nerve roots. Pain may come on suddenly after some minor knock or after bending over. The bones are so thin that such minor injury can cause a vertebra to collapse. The resulting pain is severe and can last for 6–8 weeks before it starts to improve.

Thin people are more likely to suffer from
osteoporosis, and anorexia is a real threat to
your bone density. You should aim to maintain
a reasonable body weight for your height—
giving your hips and legs a reasonable workload will help prevent osteoporosis. Go
for a diet that's rich in calcium and vitamin D. That's milk, cheese, and other dairy
foods, and canned fish particularly. Sunlight boosts vitamin D levels. And avoid
smoking or drinking too much.

Look at IDEA 32, *Hurt so bad*, for more information about pain-killing drugs.

Try another idea...

HOW DENSE ARE YOU?

The density of your bone is a measure of how solid it is. Brittle bones have a low
density. But it's not that easy to check. Scanners are costly, so it's likely that you'd
need to satisfy specific criteria to get a scan. The good news is that the radiation
dose with a DEXA scan is only a small fraction of that associated with a chest X-ray.

TREATMENTS

If you have osteoporosis and are in pain, taking painkillers regularly will enable you to
move around and stay active. Stronger drugs, such as opiates, are available if the pain
is too severe. But be careful—really strong drugs can make you a bit dreamy, and you
might be more likely to fall over and fracture something.

Treatments can include supplements of vitamin
D and calcium if you aren't getting enough in
your diet. These make hip fractures less likely
in frail elderly people. The biphosphonate

"Old age is not so bad when you consider the alternatives."
MAURICE CHEVALIER

Defining idea...

drugs stop bone from being reabsorbed. Other drugs that can be used have a hormone-like effect on your bones and are used to prevent osteoporosis, and there's also actual hormone replacement therapy, or HRT, but that's gotten bad press recently. With HRT for men, long-term risks of increased cancer of the prostate must be balanced against gains of treatment for osteoporosis.

How did it go?

Q I'm in my sixties. Should I take HRT to prevent my osteoporosis from getting worse?

A *HRT used to be advocated for women with an early menopause, or older women with a lowish bone density. Advice varies, but the risks of HRT may outweigh its benefits in slowing the thinning of your bones and preventing fractures. You'd need to take HRT for many years for it to have a significant effect. Discuss your own circumstances with your doctor.*

Q How can I avoid falling now that I'm getting older?

A *If you've got osteoporosis, the last thing you want to do is to fall and risk a fracture. Drop the sky-diving and wrestling and take up a non-contact sport instead. Exercise will improve your balance and muscle strength. Make the environments of your home and work safe. Improve your lighting, and remove rugs or other hazards lying on the floor. Are any medicines you're taking making you drowsy? If so, review them with your doctor. You can wear a hip protector—a special plastic or foam shield—on your hips to minimize risk should you take a tumble.*

38

Help me make it through the night

"You've made your bed and now you must lie on it," said one carpenter to another. For the rest of us who buy our beds, there's oodles of choice, so find one to suit your back.

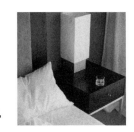

You'll spend about a third of your life in bed. So it's got to be worth investing money and effort in choosing the right one to help beat your back pain.

THE BED ITSELF

You know your bed's got to be firm and give you good support. You know that an over-soft or old mattress is *not* good. Change the mattress if you need to. Think about buying a better sprung bed or one with a wooden base. Experiment in the local bed shop until you find one that suits you and your back. Take your time—don't rush to the most snazzy bargain offer—it won't be much of a bargain if your back problems continue.

Use pillows creatively in bed, to stop yourself from rolling over if your back is really painful and an inadvertent movement is agony. Line them up against your back while lying on your side so that they wedge you in position. A pillow placed under your bent knees may help to keep you in a position that suits your back, especially if pain radiates down one of your legs. Or lie on your back with two pillows rolled within a towel placed under your knees.

Maybe you're still in the honeymoon period with your partner and don't want to sleep separately, but your back pain might be better if you could spread out instead of lying in a cramped position or hanging on to the edge of the bed. Why not have a separate bed or mattress on standby so that when you wake up in the night in pain, you can crawl off to it?

A duvet is probably more comfortable than sheets and blankets that are tucked in tightly, and it's certainly less restrictive of movement.

SLEEPING OVER AWAY FROM HOME

If you travel away from home, think of the beds you'll be staying in. If you go to a particular town as part of your work schedule, find a hotel with good beds you can depend on. Call ahead and ask about the beds or mattresses—you're the customer, don't be shy. Ask to swap rooms if faced with a hopeless mattress or bed base. Maybe the hotel staff can lift the mattress onto the floor and make up your bed there—but don't you do it and risk your back. Put a board in the trunk of your car just in case. You can bring it out to put between the bed base and soft mattress if needs be.

If you're expected to sleep on a sleeper sofa or futon, you know you'll wake up stiff and painful in the morning. So don't agree to it. Buy a deluxe air bed that promises orthopedic support. Try it out for a night first before finding you have a week ahead of you on an inadequate bed away from home and can't do anything about it.

> **A brisk walk before you go to bed may make you more comfortable at night. IDEA 7, *Keeping active*, is big on regular physical activity.**

Try another idea...

LOUNGING IN THE SUN

The sun is out, you've done the chores, and you're determined to wallow in the heat and absorb some rays. Your first challenge is getting the lounger out from the back of the shed without hurting your back. Then think. It might be comfortable to lie on for 10 minutes, but what about the 2 or 3 hours when you fall asleep? If in doubt, buy or borrow a lounger that's light enough to lift easily and strong enough to give your back support when you lay out on it asleep for hours (you hope!).

If you're away on vacation you might not have much choice—especially if you're a late riser and other guests have snagged the best loungers. If the loungers are decrepit or saggy, they are likely to make you feel the same. You might be better off lying out on the sand—making a little hollow for your body's curves. Or lie on the grass if you're not by the beach, sprawled on a thick blanket.

PILLOWS

Only you know what suits you best, but it's likely to be one or no pillow, not two or more, which would cause your neck to curve sharply when you lie down. This will pull all the way down your spine.

> *"To sleep perchance to dream."*
> WILLIAM SHAKESPEARE

Defining idea...

YOUR SLEEP ENVIRONMENT

Your back will have a better rest if you sleep well. Consider if your room is well ventilated. If it's safe to do so, open a window overnight; if it's not safe, fix bars over a small opening window and open that if necessary. But make sure you avoid drafts.

Try to cut out any external noise. Or, for that matter, noise from your partner. Get them a snoring aid if they're waking you up, or move out of the bedroom you share. Earplugs may help if you've got noisy neighbors.

How did it go?

Q **The worst time of the day when I've got a bad back is first thing in the morning. I just hate getting out of bed. Any tips (other than rolling over and going back to sleep)?**

A *Take care when getting out of bed to keep your spine in its natural alignment. Lie flat on your back with your knees bent up. Keeping your legs together, roll onto your side, at the side of the bed. Gently lower your legs over the edge of the mattress. Support yourself on your lower arm, and push yourself up with your upper arm until you reach the sitting position.*

Q **What pillows are best for my neck when that's painful as well?**

A *You can buy specially shaped pillows that support the nape of your neck. Look at a catalog in a pharmacy or on the Internet to see the varieties offered. In an emergency, roll up a small towel to a sausage shape to go underneath a slim pillow to support your neck.*

39

Give it a break

You owe it to yourself to have a good vacation. With the price of travel, you'll owe it to the bank, too.

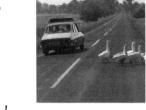

Watch out, there are hundreds of risks around—when you go away from home and your normal routine.

You work hard, and you need a good break to relax and recover from all the pressures on you. It might be jetting off to the sun, an active break, or simply spending time at home, but the mental break and time for doing exercise and sports should help your back.

GETTING YOUR LUGGAGE THERE

If you're taking hand luggage on a train or plane, buy one with wheels like airline pilots use (that's the luggage, not the plane). Choose your suitcases carefully. Even if they have wheels, you'll still have to lift them onto the train, into the trunk of the car, onto the airport luggage rack. Go for two small suitcases rather than one big, heavy one—divide and conquer. The wheels should be a reasonable size and turn easily even when your case is loaded. The case should be designed so that it's easy to push or maneuver. Don't get distracted by the children squabbling or time pressures—concentrate on lifting your cases in a way that avoids straining your

Here's an idea for you...
Get the timing right. Book travel times that mean you're not sitting on the train or plane overnight, even if that means missing some peak sunbathing time. Conversely, if you're going by car, leave before dawn to cut your journey time by half.

back. You don't want your view of the Mediterranean to be your hotel ceiling as you lie flat on your back, unable to leave your room.

Take plenty of small bills for tipping the porters. They want to carry your cases and you don't want to hurt your back—it's a win–win situation.

SITTING COMFORTABLY

When sitting for a long time in a train or plane, get up and walk around as often as you can. If you change trains or planes or they're delayed, go walk—don't just sit and wait. Don't drop off to sleep in a contorted position—choose a window seat so you can lean against the side. Carry a shaped neck rest and use that to keep you in an upright position.

BE A REAL SPORT

If you're usually inactive at home, try to incorporate some physical activity into your vacation. Walking, cycling, and swimming are all great for your back. Any exercise that strengthens your back without twisting it will be right for you, so go sailing, rowing, or skiing (just don't fall down a mountain). If you do a sport that's new to you or for which you're out of practice, take it easy

Try another idea...
Look at IDEA 11, *Take a stand or sit tight*, for tips on comfort when you're sitting for long periods.

at first. Pace yourself and build up the time you spend on it over successive days. Any sport involving a ball will require you to strike out powerfully with one side of your body (like soccer or tennis) or twist your back (like golf). Beware, because sometimes you only find out you've overdone things the next day, when you wake up, stiff and in pain, with your vacation ruined.

You can still exercise while on the move. Look at IDEA 20, *At the core of the matter*, to read about the benefits of Pilates exercises.

...and another

LIFT OFF

If your idea of a vacation is decorating at home, don't be lured into thinking your "nest" is safe—danger lurks around every corner. Think how you lift—those stepladders, cans of paint, shifting furniture out of the way. Invest in some scaffolding to let you stand on two feet, facing the job straight. Don't stand precariously on a rickety chair, use proper steps. Choose steps with a handle at the top to hold on to.

"I have never taken any exercise except sleeping and resting."
MARK TWAIN

Defining idea...

If your dream vacation is transforming the garden, it'll be a nightmare if you hurt your back digging up tangled old bushes on the first day. Mix hard and easy jobs so you use different muscles. Build up to the task by working in the garden for a few evenings before the blitz on the weeds. Use equipment that is suitable for your jobs. Maybe a new fork or spade might make digging easier to do and will require less brute strength.

"Everyone dies, but not everyone lives."
A. SACHS, author

Defining idea...

173

How did it go?

Q **I like to spend my vacation in art galleries and museums, but all that standing around makes my back ache. Should I sacrifice my love of art and settle for an activity vacation instead to keep my back in shape?**

A   *If you've spent much of the day looking at art galleries or having retail therapy in shopping centers, a brisk two-mile walk should counterbalance all that standing. Schedule your walks in at lunchtime and in the evenings. You'll see a lot more of the town or country you're visiting if you walk around rather than whiz past in a bus, taxi, or car, too.*

Q **I want to book a family vacation with something for everyone. But as a single parent I seem to spend all my time pandering to my overactive children. How can I prioritize what I want?**

A   *Choose a hotel or campsite with a health club and swimming pool. See if there are some complementary therapies to try. If there's a babysitting or child-care facility, you can go to the gym or have therapy while the kids are otherwise engaged. Book a place where the kids can use the equipment, too, so you can all join in. The staff at the health club will encourage a healthy lifestyle and you'll leave feeling lots better as well as having strengthened your back through the activities there.*

40

A day in your life

Escape to a health spa and become one of the health brigade. But don't fool yourself into thinking you're resting. They'll have you working up a sweat quicker than you can say "white dressing gown."

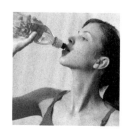

You should find lots of different activities (and other guests with well-toned bodies!) to tempt you down at the health spa.

It could be just what you need—a day at the health spa. Start by sending for the brochure and working out your program for the day, so you can book some of your activities in advance. You don't want to be disappointed when you get there.

COMPLEMENTARY THERAPIES

You can't go to a health spa without trying one or two of these. Experience at least one hands-on treatment. Whether you try massage or aromatherapy, be sure to tell the practitioner about your back problem so that they can tailor their treatment to your needs. It's your chance to experiment with a therapy you haven't tried before. Organize the treatments for after you've had the most strenuous exercise, so you can rest, relax, and recover. Don't undo all the good the complementary therapy has done by frantic exercise in the gym afterward.

Here's an idea for you... **If the health spa has a flotation chamber—that's a tank filled with saltwater to help you float, with no light, no sound, and no distractions—give it a try. You just lie there, with your senses suspended. After a spell there your back should feel great (so long as you don't suffer from claustrophobia!).**

PLENTY OF EXERCISE

The swimming pool may have a hydrotherapy area with a Jacuzzi, where jets of water pummel your poor back, increasing the circulation with their massaging effect. Try the massage chairs that you can sit in after your swim. Going with a group of friends can be fun as you encourage one another to try the various pieces of equipment. But choose the friends wisely—you don't want them showing you up with their svelte, hard bodies!

There are probably bicycles you can use to explore the grounds or go farther afield to explore the local roads. Riding in the grounds means you won't have to worry about traffic, leaving you free to enjoy the fresh air and the countryside or garden flowers—ah, bliss!

Use the opportunity to try activities you don't usually do because of lack of time or facilities. You might be able to play croquet or try archery to improve the flexibility of your upper trunk. Join in tennis or squash if the health club pairs off players or organizes matches. There might be off-site activities such as horse riding or quad biking—all involving muscles you don't usually use.

BEAUTY TREATMENTS

Get a makeover to lift your spirits. If you have your hair done, be careful when it's being washed if your back's painful. It's probably better to bend your head backward into the basin, keeping your back extended, rather than slumping forward. Let the hairdresser know what suits your back— don't be forced into a painful position.

You may try the sunbeds and the heat will feel lovely on your back, but don't expose yourself for too long or your sunburn will cause havoc in bed later.

Once you've sampled different kinds of complementary therapies at the health spa, find out where you can continue with your favorites when you're back at home. IDEA 12, *What's the alternative?*, will give you lots of options.

Try another idea...

SOAK UP THE ATMOSPHERE

If you've got any bad habits—smoking, drinking heavily, being inactive, overeating— then make up your mind to change your behavior and change it forever. You may have felt guilty about your "little weakness" for some time and even made several resolutions to change—only to relapse. What better place to learn more about how to change and see the benefits of a healthy lifestyle than at the health spa? Let your day there be the first day of the rest of your life, where you eat a healthy diet, take regular and varied exercise, relax and enjoy yourself, don't smoke cigarettes, and drink alcohol only in moderation. Hmmm, yes, perhaps that is asking a bit much. But at least make a start and improve your lifestyle in a staged way.

Swap health tips with others at the health spa, and watch how they use the gym equipment. Learn from them and try their ways yourself.

"If God had wanted me to touch my toes, he would've put chocolate on the floor!"
BEV (cartoon)

Defining idea...

177

How did it go?

Q **I can't get away and indulge myself at a health spa when there's so much to do at home with the children and all. Can I?**

A *What about persuading the boss that the local health spa is just the place for a team retreat? Then you'd have the best of both worlds. You could go on work time and needn't feel guilty about neglecting the kids. And after you've done some work to justify being there, you could try out the beauty treatments and facilities with your friends. If the boss doesn't fall for it, get on the phone—I'm sure Grandma would love to look after your "little darlings."*

Q **A day at a health spa sounds great, but it's over too quickly, isn't it?**

A *Take a camera and get someone to take pictures of you doing lots of different activities there. Put a picture on your fridge or as a screensaver on your PC to remind you of the fun you had and as a prompt to do more exercise. Fill in a postcard at the health spa with your new resolutions and ask a friend to mail it to you in three months' time. What a shock you'll get when your postcard arrives in the mail reminding you of all those promises you've been faithfully keeping ever since!*

41

Everything's coming up roses

Don't dig a hole for yourself by making your back pain worse when you're gardening. Find ways to weed and dig without straining your back.

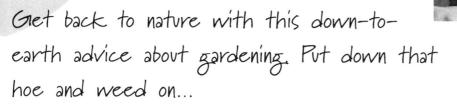

Get back to nature with this down-to-earth advice about gardening. Put down that hoe and weed on...

READY, STEADY, GO

Do some gentle stretching before you start gardening. Then, when you're out there, intersperse lighter tasks with heavy digging to give your back a breather. Don't do heavy digging for more than 10–20 minutes at a time.

Bend your knees rather than your back when digging or weeding. Exert any force through your knees and thighs, using your arms and shoulders as a secondary force. Whenever possible, use a kneeler or knee pads rather than bend over. Keep close to a tree or shrub that you're pulling out. Be careful not to jerk suddenly to pull plants out or twist while you are tugging on their roots.

179

Sit down on a small stool to do the weeding so that you keep your back straight. Choose a stool with runners along the base rather than legs that sink into soft ground. If you can weed your borders from a path or paved driveway, the stool could be on castors—then you can scoot up and down to reach the far-flung weeds.

EASY PEASY

Move or carry several small loads rather than shift one large one. You could put heavy tubs on castors to make them easier to move around. If you're looking to gravel or mulch with a few economy-sized 25 lb bags from the garden center, don't let your financial savings be at the expense of your back. Get the guys in the center to load up the car and have them stand the bags upright, not lay them flat— they'll be at waist height and easier to lift out when you get home. At home, set a wheelbarrow by the side of the car and lift the bags out carefully with your knees bent and back straight. That way you'll minimize the drop.

TIDY DOES IT

Keep your shed or garage tidy so that you don't have to risk your back reaching over piles of junk for those essential tools. Be careful not to overreach yourself when lifting the lids of cold frames. Use lightweight plastic sheeting so that the lid is light to lift, or rig up a pulley and counterbalance to make it easier to manage.

REST-OR-ACTION

Place a well-made seat in the garden for rests. Make sure that it has a firm backrest and is not too low for you to sit comfortably with your feet flat on the ground. Put it in a sheltered corner of the garden to avoid drafts.

CHOOSE THE RIGHT TOOLS

Use long-handled lightweight tools so you can keep your back straight and lighten the load on your arms. Check that your tools suit you for their weight, height, and balance. Earth clings less to stainless steel forks and spades than to carbon steel ones, making the weight you're lifting less. Use a spade with a small blade rather than a full-sized digging spade so you're not tempted to lift too much soil at a time.

A two-wheeled wheelbarrow with a stroller-type handle requires less effort to push than other kinds. A suction tool for clearing up leaves is easier on your back than raking and shoveling. Get an easy-to-work hosepipe and attachments so that you aren't carrying watering cans or buckets of water. If you do use cans, place water butts strategically around your garden to minimize the distance you have to carry the water. Buy an electric hedge trimmer so you don't have to use hand shears.

IDEA 6, *Ooh, you don't want to do that...*, emphasizes some good techniques for when you're lifting.

Try another idea...

"The man who would call a spade a spade should be compelled to use one. It is the only thing he is fit for."
OSCAR WILDE

Defining idea...

CHANGE THE LAYOUT OF YOUR GARDEN

Go for raised beds so you don't have to stoop to garden. Limit the width of your borders so that you can reach across them easily without stretching too far. Plant shrubs and ground cover plants rather than annual bedding plants, so there's less to do in the garden but it still looks good. Go for plants that don't need regular watering even in a hot summer.

Replace your lawn with a paved area so that you don't have to mow the grass or empty the grass container. Alternatively, grass over any plant beds and extend your lawn. In a dry summer let grass cuttings lie, so that the lawn mower's lighter and easier to maneuver. Opt for an electric mower if possible. If you have a gas mower, start it up by bracing one foot against the machine for balance, then pull the cord.

How did it go?

Q   I love working in my greenhouse. My tomatoes are to die for, but murder on my back. How can I pot my plants in my greenhouse more comfortably?

A   *Make sure that the workbenches in your greenhouse are at the right height. They need to be 2–4 inches below the height of your elbow so that you don't have to bend. Get a high stool so that you can sit comfortably at the bench while doing your potting. Playing music might help you relax, too—and could do wonders for your pelargoniums.*

Q   I think hanging baskets are head and shoulders above other patio containers, but they're not easy to manage. Any tips?

A   *Put hanging baskets in light shade so you have to water them less often. If you get a hanging basket sprayer, you won't have to hold your watering can above head height. Planting in special compost with moisture-retaining crystals will again mean less watering. Buy a pulley attachment so that you can lower and raise the baskets with ease.*

42

Driving force

In, out, in, out, and shake it all about—and if your car's a good one your back will stand up to that sort of rough handling.

No one car will suit everyone. Make sure yours suits your body size and shape. If you must travel in other people's cars, you need to adapt them for max comfort.

BUYING A CAR

When you take a car for a test drive, don't just think about the way it handles around corners, or whether you like the sunroof or other gadgets. Think about the seating and how it suits you. You need a car where you can sit comfortably on seating that helps you to maintain a good posture. Try to take the car for a reasonably long drive so that you can see how comfortable you are after 20 or 30 minutes; a quick spin around the block is about as informative as a glass of water.

Here's an idea for you...

Avoid using your car as an office. If you're early for a meeting, don't use your laptop in the car or sort out papers there—you'll just get into cramped positions or end up twisting across to the backseat to pick up papers. Better to sit in the foyer of the place you're visiting and work there.

MAKING ADJUSTMENTS

The more adjustable features there are in the car seating, the more likely it is to suit your needs. Take your time to adjust the position of the seat before you set off so that you can reach the steering wheel and pedals comfortably without stretching. Check that you can fully depress the clutch and accelerator pedals. Make sure that the car seat is firm and gives you good support for your back and thighs. The seat should be wider than your hips and thighs, and the backrest wide enough to support your shoulders. Look for a seat where you can adjust the height and tilt independently of each other. See if there's a built-in height adjustment if you're short or tall. Adjust the seat so that it leans back slightly and is comfortable for your back and neck. Find out if the angle of the steering wheel can be altered, or if it can move up and down, to create a more comfortable position for your arms and give you clearance when you operate the floor pedals. Make sure the seat will move back far enough to allow your legs and arms to be in a relaxed, slightly bent position. There should be a space between the edge of your seat and your knees to allow for movement and to prevent your circulation from being cut off.

After you've finished making all these adjustments you should be able to reach all the hand controls easily and have a good view of the display instruments on the dashboard. Make sure that you have maximum vision of the roads and surroundings outside the car. The backrest should give support along the length of your back to shoulder height but should not obstruct your rear vision. You should be able to sit upright with plenty of headroom. If you're going to be carrying several passengers on a regular basis, how's the seating for their backs?

Insist on power steering, which will make maneuvering easier with less strain on your back. Consider buying an automatic car so that you have fewer pedal movements to do.

GETTING OUT OF THE CAR

If you're going to be transporting heavy weights as shopping or as part of your work, choose a car with a suitable trunk. You'll want to be able to lift any loads into and out of the trunk with a good posture that minimizes any strain on your back as described in IDEA 4, *Hold your head up high*, and IDEA 6, *Ooh, you don't want to do that...*

Try another idea...

Get out of your car without twisting your back. Move your whole body toward the door, keeping your thighs together. Then slide your body around by 90 degrees to place your feet together on the ground outside the car and stand up. You can actually buy a revolving car seat that will save you the struggle when getting in or out of the car.

Don't bend to unload the trunk right after driving a long distance—limber up first with a few exercises to stretch your back. Hold any load as close to your body as possible as you lift it. Don't lift and twist at the same time. Face forward, square to the load you're lifting. Don't twist around to pick up bags from the backseat when you're in the front. Get out, open the back door, and lift the bags out from there instead.

"To travel hopefully is a better thing than to arrive."
ROBERT LOUIS STEVENSON

Defining idea...

185

How did
it go?

Q **I guess I'm impatient. When I travel, I like to get to point B in minimum time with minimum fuss. But when I do, I emerge from my car like a rolled-up hedgehog. How often should I take a break on a long journey, back-wise?**

A *Think of stopping for up to 15 minutes every 2 hours that you've been driving. However comfortable your car seating is, you'll still need to take regular breaks from driving to stretch and change position. Readjust your seating position when you stop if you're uncomfortable. Go for a brisk walk for a few minutes.*

Q **I've adjusted the seating in my car but I still get uncomfy on long drives. Is there anything else I can try?**

A *Try a wedge or thin cushion under your buttocks to raise your hips to be level with your knees. Some cars have an adjustable lumbar support incorporated into the car seat. Increasing the support exaggerates the curve of the seat to fit the shape of your lower back. If your car doesn't have this, using a lumbar roll can maintain you in a good sitting position with a hollow in your back.*

43

Mom's the word

Milk being pregnant as much as possible to get out of lifting or doing anything else you'd rather not do. Go for the "help me" pity vote and you can sit it out for nine months.

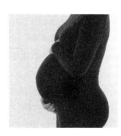

Prepare your body for pregnancy by building up a strong and flexible back before you even conceive. That'll be regular physical activity and sports, or opt for specific exercise programs for moms-to-be.

YOUR BODY AND PREGNANCY

Once you're pregnant, the ligaments of your spine become more lax due to increased levels of hormones circulating around your body. This allows your pelvis to expand during labor so that you can give birth. It also means that the joints of your spine and how the spine attaches to your pelvic bone may become unstable. The ligaments may remain lax for several months after you've had the baby, so be careful not to overstretch your back muscles once the baby's been born, too.

Here's an idea for you...

Try Pilates before you get pregnant. Pilates exercises can help you to build up strong pelvic and abdominal muscles, and strengthen your back for pregnancy. You'll want to be sure that all your internal organs are well positioned with well toned muscles to resist the pressures as the baby grows and you start to bulge.

Your abdominal muscles will be stretched over a progressively larger expanse as your baby grows. During pregnancy the two halves of your rectus abdominis—the muscles that run down the front of your stomach—separate to allow the uterus to grow larger. To stay in shape you'll need to gently exercise your abdominal muscles. However, you won't be focusing on strengthening them, as they need to be reasonably relaxed to let your uterus expand and the baby move around.

Your breasts will enlarge and their heaviness might drag your shoulders forward, causing your upper spine to curve more. So invest in a good bra that supports you well and helps you to keep your shoulders straight with your spine in its natural position.

Pilates exercises are not recommended before 14 weeks of pregnancy, when you're more at risk of miscarrying. After that, you'll have to experiment with the types of positions for exercising that suit you. Lying on your back will be out if it triggers heartburn. You might find the relaxation exercises really helpful after a hard day at work. Not only can they help you get through your pregnancy, they can also help you regain your strength and flexibility after your postnatal check when the baby's six weeks old.

AFTER THE BABE'S BORN

Your pelvic floor muscles lose all sense of purpose and condition during pregnancy, so if you want to avoid incontinence and go running without wetting yourself or having to wear a diaper, concentrate on strengthening those muscles. Pelvic floor exercises are at the core of the Pilates exercise program, but you can get a leaflet from your OB/GYN describing the movements to do.

The key to a comfy back is...posture, posture, posture. Lying on a firm bed and sitting in good supportive chairs will be even more important than usual when you're pregnant. Your back will need all the support it can get, as your tummy is pulling for two. Look at IDEA 38, *Help me make it through the night*, for advice on beds.

Try another idea...

Do lots of general physical activity. Start walking, biking, or swimming again after a few weeks. Get someone to look after the baby so that you can have dedicated, regular time to exercise and get fit. This will help you to work off any excess weight you've accumulated during pregnancy, and regain your feeling of well-being if you had a tough labor or first few weeks. Your back should start to get stronger and your abs should begin to tighten up, so you get back to a flatter stomach.

It's easy to forget to do postnatal exercises once the baby's born and you're screamingly busy. If you can't make time, do them whenever you're at the sink washing up, preparing your baby's bottles, or cleaning their babywear (i.e., most of the time!). Contract those muscles, hold for a count of ten, and relax. Repeat ten times and try and do the sequence three times a day. You know that you've got the right muscles if you can stop yourself urinating in mid-flow, or at least constrict the flow.

"The cock croweth but the hen delivereth the goods."
ANONYMOUS

Defining idea...

189

LIFTING

Be careful how you lift during pregnancy, what with your lax joints and new center of gravity as your expanding uterus pulls you forward. After the birth, think about your back when you're lifting the baby and his paraphernalia, even if the baby's crying and you're distracted. Don't lift the baby into the car seat in the back of the car without doing your best to avoid twisting your back or overstretching. Don't lift an older child and the baby at the same time. Make allowances for the baby's wriggling so he doesn't jerk your spine in an unexpected way.

How did it go?

Q   I look like a whale, I vomit every morning, and now I have a dreadful backache! Is it an unavoidable fact of pregnancy?

A   *As your baby grows and your uterus bulges, you'll tend to stand with your back hollowed. You may even find yourself putting both hands on your waist and arching backward, as pregnant women seem to take up this stance unconsciously. But this position stresses your lumbar spine, so the more basic exercise you do that strengthens your low back, the better. You could also try a supportive corset from a maternity clothes shop to see if that will restore your back to a more comfortable position, though don't wear it all the time.*

Q   What's the best exercise for a lazy slob like me who hasn't really thought about getting in shape until I got pregnant?

A   *If you haven't been keeping in shape, don't suddenly go crazy exercising once you find that you're pregnant. Start with brisk walking and work up slowly to doing more activities involving specific parts of your body, or just go for longer walks.*

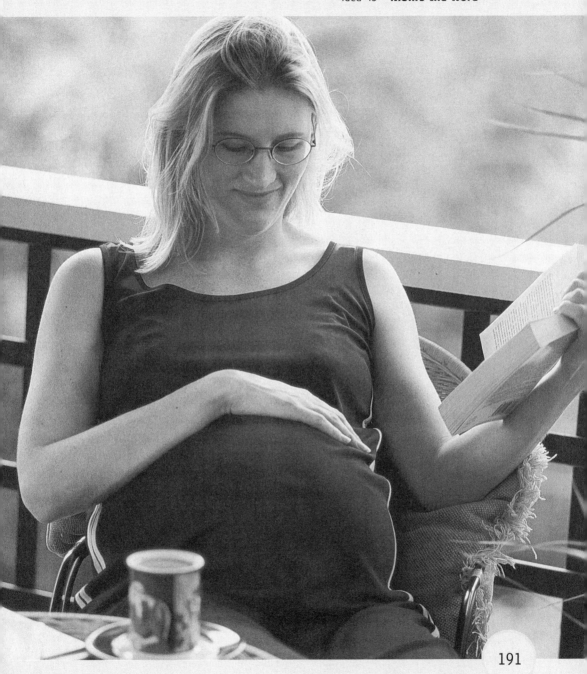

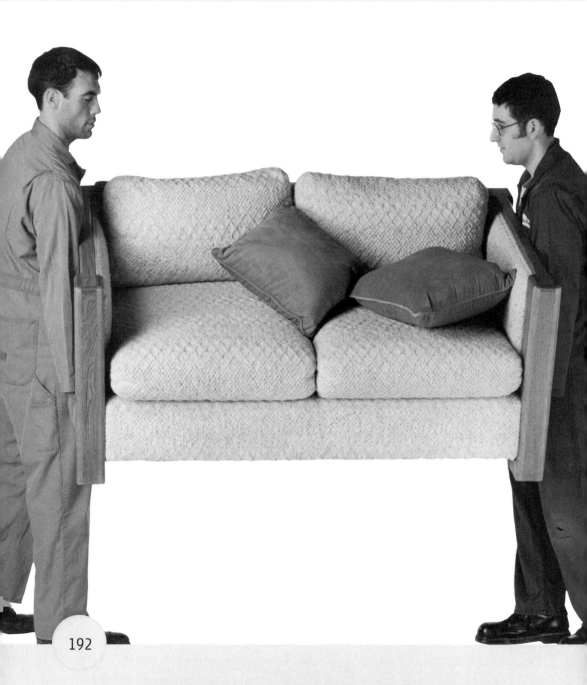

44

Wish you were there

The moving van pulls up at your new pad—where risks are waiting to happen. There's carrying her over the threshold, assembling her gigantic wardrobe as utmost priority so her clothes don't get crushed, adjusting the big-screen TV for her well-earned rest...

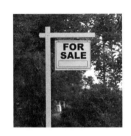

Start planning for a move well in advance so you come through with your back unscathed.

GET THE RIGHT HELP

Can you get a team of people together to help you move house? Besides all the legal and financial paperwork, you need help to pack up your possessions, tidy the garden and garage, clean your old house and the new one if necessary, transport your goods, unload, unpack, and perhaps redecorate—phew! That's a lot of risks for an iffy back. But you don't have to do it all—delegate as much as you can, or can afford. Factor in money for employing help when you're calculating the costs of the move.

Here's an idea for you...

Call a family meeting and agree on who's doing what as soon as you know the move's on. Don't wait for the contract to be signed—start preparing once you have a verbal agreement. Get everyone in the house to review what needs to be packed up and taken to the new house and what can be disposed of beforehand.

LIFTING FURNITURE

Those rules about lifting maximum weights at work apply just as much when you're at home, even if there's no health and safety inspector with clipboard watching nearby. You'll be lifting objects of all sorts of sizes and shapes. Think where the center of gravity is first, then move around it so that you lift it with its center of gravity next to you.

Buy a trolley to move heavy furniture. Make sure it's robust enough for big items and that you can maneuver it easily. Even if you employ movers to move your belongings to your new house, you'll still want to move single items of furniture about as you find their best position.

Try to pack a mix of object types in each box—so only half fill it with heavy books before topping it off with lighter, bulkier items. Label whether a box is light, heavy, or very heavy after you've packed it—so anyone picking it up is forewarned.

Don't move more furniture than you have to. If you have surplus furniture, sell it or give it to charity, making it clear that the lucky recipient collects. Put any unwanted items you'll be taking to the charity stores in small boxes of manageable weight that are stored at waist height, so that you avoid unnecessary stooping and lifting from low levels. Review what you've got in the garage and the attic, too, not just in the house itself—it's all got to go. Dispose of your unwanted or surplus belongings well before the actual move date so that you spread the lifting and carrying over a number of weeks, rather than just a few days of frenzied activity.

SHARING THE LOAD

See if a friend will help you dig up any precious plants you want to take with you. If their back is strong, ask them to empty the attic or carry your possessions up from the basement. (If they're really strong, perhaps they could carry you, too.) If you're doing these jobs, remember about sensible lifting, keeping your back straight and knees bent. Take care not to overbalance while carrying heavy or bulky items down the steps from the attic. If possible, lower the heavy items down using carpet webbing or a rope. God made gravity (or was it Isaac Newton?), so use it. If there are two of you lifting together, take care to spread the weight fairly. Discuss and agree how you'll both lift and carry together, so that one of you isn't suddenly left taking all the weight while the other walks in front, opening doors, and so forth.

DON'T OVERREACH YOURSELF

When you're getting curtains down, or putting them up, use stepladders so that you're not reaching above your head to take the weight of the curtains. You can then loop the curtains over the top of the stepladders so that you're not carrying their full weight while you continue unhooking them.

If you've got a piano or heavy gym equipment, you might want to pay for professionals to move it, even if you're managing the rest of the move yourself. But if you're doing it all, then get friends and family to help and use a cart.

Don't rush the cleaning. There may be years of dirt under some of your furniture, like the washing machine or the piano. IDEA 9, *Full scream ahead*, gives hints for lots of different chores.

Try another idea...

"You've got to be a nutcase to do this. The best bit is when it's all over."
PRINCE PHILIP

Defining idea...

195

How did
it go?

**Q We've hired a van and are moving ourselves to save money. There
are some pretty steep steps leading up to the front door of our
new house. Any tips on getting our stuff into the house?**

A *When you get to your new house, see if you can back up the van, then
position a ramp from the back door of the van to the front door of your
new house, bridging the steps up to it. That'll save you from having to walk
up the steps carrying heavy loads. You'll have to think this out well in
advance so you can put the ramp together.*

**Q Any tips for lifting large objects, like the fridge or dresser, so as
not to hurt ourselves?**

A *Get a length of carpet webbing or similar strapping so you're not
overreaching awkwardly around a large object like a fridge. If two people
each take an end, they can synchronize the lift and share the load, then
carry it along on a cart. You can lift and lower a dresser down a flight of
stairs like that fairly easily (in theory anyway!). Oh, and don't forget to
empty them first.*

45

Listening in

You can learn a lot from other people—even if it's the "do as I say and not as I do" type of advice.

You'll find lots of people peddling advice to get on your bike and cycle to work. And they've got a point: Cycling will get your joints in gear if you put your back into it.

Listening to other people's stories will extend your range of ideas, and some of their tips might be just right for you, too. If you watch the way other people do things at work or when you're out and about, you might spot good gadgets or techniques to help you lift or do awkward jobs. Here are some ideas that you might pick up.

PUT UP WITH THE PAIN?

Some people swear that taking painkillers or anti-inflammatory drugs lets them stay active and go to work as usual. Other people prefer to put up with the pain so that they know how their back is doing, and can adjust their movements to minimize the strain that they feel they're putting on their back. No one is right or wrong—you can opt for either approach.

Choose a hobby that works for you. If your friends egg you on to join them in their favorite sport, be it karate, ice skating, or bowling, and you find it keeps your back strong and flexible, unlike the golf or tennis you used to play, then go for it.

MAKING EXERCISE A HABIT

Chatting to other people, you'll find they all have their favorite exercise sequence. One of your friends might tell you about how he stands on a circular disc, keeping his feet still, and does gentle rotating movements of his trunk to soothe his back pain and get rid of his stiffness. Background music might be the way that other people keep their exercise session going without getting bored or giving up. If you join a sports club or get onto a team you'll feel obliged to turn up regularly, even when you're feeling lazy—and that'll help keep you motivated.

IT'S OKAY TO BE A LOSER

Lose the car. You may not have the sort of job to be able to do that if you live a long way from work, visit clients decked out in a business suit, or carry loads around as part of your job. But so long as you're safe on the roads, cycling or walking to work's a good idea for introducing more exercise into your working day.

ASK AN OLD GUY HOW HE'S KEPT SO FIT

It won't take much encouragement to get older people telling you what they do to keep fit. So ask one or two who are spry for their age about their routines (wait until you've plenty of time to listen to the answers!). It could be an early morning

"The only thing to do with good advice is to pass it on. It is never any use to oneself."
OSCAR WILDE

exercise routine of touching their toes then standing up 30 times before they shower and have breakfast. They may do simple back-stretching exercises to limber up their lumbar spine—like lying flat on their back with their arms stretched out and crossing one leg over the other as far as it will go, then repeating it with the other leg. They may walk several miles a day or play golf several times a week—which is the same thing, but with some swinging movements thrown in for good measure.

If you want to get more exercise, look up IDEA 7, _Keeping active_. A personal trainer recommended by a friend could advise you about the best exercises for your back, how to use gym equipment safely, and what activities to avoid.

Try another idea...

LEARN WHAT NOT TO DO

This is a difficult one. Listen to other people's warnings of what triggered their back pain and avoid it yourself. Take heed from people whose back "went" when they were doing sit-ups. When you hear of people's trips, slips, and falls, double-check your home or office to make sure you won't fall for the same thing. When you see older people doing sports or activities that are beyond them and putting their backs at risk, such as competitive squash or mountaineering, learn their lesson for them and stop doing that activity yourself before you reach the same age bracket. Watch people lift, and consider how you'd do it differently if it looks awkward. And don't be afraid to offer your own advice, either.

"To know the road ahead ask those coming back."
CHINESE PROVERB

Defining idea...

Q **Enough already! All this advice—I don't know where to start first! What do you suggest?**

A   *You can't always believe what other people tell you, and what works for them won't necessarily work for you. But if you've still got back pain despite all the ideas you've been trying, you might as well try following their tips. At least you'll have somebody to blame if it all goes wrong!*

Q **It's great to know the huge range of things I can do to help my back pain. Last time my back pain came on out of the blue I was really stuck as I couldn't remember how I'd beaten it before. Yes, I know that's pretty dumb, but I wasn't planning on it happening again. What's the answer?**

A   *Write down your plan in case it happens again. When you wake up one morning and can't move, you'll have something to remind you what to do. Cover exercises that work for you, maybe doing push-ups without raising your bottom from the ground. Try ice or heat packs—have some ready. Describe the best position for propping yourself up in bed to ease the pain with the specific arrangement of your pillows that works for you. Include the telephone number of a trusted physiotherapist, or maybe the contact details for a chiropractor or osteopath.*

46

Play it safe at home

"Safety first" sounds dull. But if you trip or slip and really hurt your back, it will be duller still just lying around for days on end.

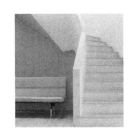

Walk around your home to spot any hazards that could trigger back pain if you were careless or unlucky. Now don't just stand there—do something about them!

PREVENT TRIPS OR SLIPS

Look for loose rugs in the hallway, living room, or bedrooms. Could you catch your foot under the edge of the rug, sending you flying? Or if you walk quickly over the rug, will it slip on the shiny floor underneath, depositing you unceremoniously on your bottom with a thump, jarring your back in the fall? If so, get rid of the rug, and if it was covering up a stain or worn carpet, put up with that or replace it.

Are there objects left lying around that you could trip over, perhaps children's toys or maybe ornaments? Move them now and make sure everyone keeps them out of the way of the walk-through areas of your house.

Think services. Store your trash in smaller bags so you can lift them easily. Get a wheeled trashcan if you don't already have one and keep it near the back door so you don't have far to carry your trash bags. If you get groceries delivered, place a shelf or cupboard outside your front door, so that neither you nor the deliveryman has to stoop to ground level to handle the goods. Raise your mailbox up if it's near the ground and put a box or shelf inside the front door to catch the mail or your newspaper.

See if there's more you can do to make the steps or stairs in your home safer. Is the handrail on your stairs robust enough to let you pull on it? Is it firmly attached to the wall? You could add a handrail to any outside steps up to your house, which will help in the winter when it's icy. Have a sack of sand standing by in your garage (or hall) in winter for scattering on the steps when the temperature falls after dark.

LOOK AT YOUR LIGHTING

If your place is well lit you'll be less likely to trip over objects left lying around inside your home or outside in the grounds. Check out your drive and garden paths to ensure that there are no loose flagstones or uneven paving stones to trip you.

REVIEW YOUR FURNITURE

Look at your chairs and beds with fresh eyes. Do they still give you good support or have their springs sprung their last? If you can't afford to replace them perhaps you can repair them, or buy wedges of hard foam to refresh the seat cushions or alter their angles. A hard board under a mattress that's seen better days should prevent some of the sagging when you lie on it.

What about when visitors come to stay? If you intend to give up your bed, consider where you'll be sleeping. If it's a sofa bed, check whether the mattress is suitable for an adult or really only supports the weight of a child, and replace it if necessary.

When working at your desk at home, check that you have good posture. See IDEA 5, *Ergonomics—pure science*, for a reminder.

Try another idea...

If you work on a computer from home, check that you can sit comfortably at your desk or table. Don't have lower standards for your study at home than you have for your office at work, especially if you spend an hour or more at a time working there.

Look in the kitchen and check the height of your work surface. If it's too low, can you organize a moveable raised surface so that you can work at your own waist height when doing kitchen chores like preparing a meal?

MULTI-STORAGE

Try to avoid storing heavy items at ground level or at the back of closets. Otherwise you'll be lifting heavy weights unnecessarily or reaching for them over other objects and twisting as you lift them. Instead, build shelves at various heights in your storage closets or in the garage. Or buy bookshelves to put in the utility room or an empty bedroom. Although you might save a little money bulk-buying massive quantities of food and cleaning fluids, buy smaller quantities for easier lifting.

"You've got to make a conscious decision every day to shed the old—whatever 'the old' means for you."
SARAH BAN BREATHNACH, author

Defining idea...

203

How did it go? **Q** **There are some jobs at home where you just can't eliminate all the risks, aren't there? Like washing the outside of upstairs windows.**

A *If you can't pay someone else to do it, consider how you could be safer if using a ladder outside. If you're washing upstairs windows, you could tie your ladder to one of the struts of the window frame or hammer a strong nail into the outside of the window frame to tie it onto. Alternatively, there's a gadget you can buy to wash your windows so that the sponge on the outside is magnetized to another one inside and mirrors the washing movements you make from inside. So you wash the inside and outside for half the effort—perfect!*

Q **We're about to redecorate our house. Got any tips on how to make sure I don't strain my back?**

A *Rent an electric wallpaper scraper rather than stripping wallpaper entirely by hand. Use a paintbrush with a long pole for putting on paint above head height, to avoid stretching and reaching too far. Make sure the steps you use are stable, and resist the temptation to stand on a box rather than getting the steps out just because you can't be bothered. Hold a decorating party: Invite half a dozen friends and family and offer them pizza and beer— but only when the work's done.*

47

Play it safe at work

If there's a rush job, think of yourself first, and don't break your back just to boost the boss's bonus.

The risks to you will depend on the nature of your work and how varied it is. But there are rules for these things, you know.

KNOW YOUR LIMITATIONS

Be confident in your ability to do a job. Don't go beyond that, even if instructed by your boss or egged on by your friends. You know how far you can climb up the ladder and still feel safe and able to get the job done. Health and safety regs are there to protect you. So if the forklift is not around or it's broken, don't agree to do much heavier lifting than usual just because you're told to. You're likely to strain your back and may end up taking a sick leave, which'll be much more inconvenient to them at work in the long run.

As you get older you have to accept that you can't do what you did when you were younger (so no more grumping, then!). You won't be able to lift such heavy weights or work for so long without a break once you're in your forties and older. Don't feel you're losing face when the youngsters get more done. It's not a competition and, with your experience, you'll probably achieve more in different ways.

Here's an idea for you...

Wear the right shoes for your job. If you're likely to be outdoors you'll need shoes with a deep tread to give you a good grip when walking and climbing over slippery surfaces. Even inside jobs require rubber soles so you don't slip if there's lots of water around. If you move in fashionable circles, don't walk around in very high heeled shoes as these force your spine into stressful positions. Insoles might help maintain the curve of your spine if you've got flat feet.

BE PREPARED

Read the manuals before you operate any machines or heavy equipment. Don't assume you can work them without learning all about them first. Otherwise you might get something caught in the machine or need to jerk it into action if it gets stuck, possibly hurting your back.

Be prepared for any eventuality at work that might put your back at risk. For instance, if you're out traveling and get stuck in the snow, have you got a blanket in the trunk to go under your wheels or a snow shovel to make it easier to get your car going? Have you got a set of jumper cables to jump-start your or someone else's car in the event of a dead battery? A mini-toolset in your handbag or briefcase might help you to open or repair something with minimal effort without jerking your back. Know where to go for backup or advice if a job is too much for you—don't struggle alone.

GUARDING AGAINST ATTACK

Violence at work is more common than we like to think. Woundings, common assault, robbery, and snatch theft can happen at work, the same as they can in the street—or even at home. It's more likely with some jobs than others. Nurses are particularly vulnerable, for instance. They are in close contact with people who are mentally ill, when patients or relatives can suddenly become irrational or aggressive. If you visit people in their own homes as a salesperson or to carry out a repair job, be constantly aware of the potential danger to your personal safety. Traveling alone in cars, especially in the dark, increases your risk of being attacked.

All the sensible advice applies to you at work. That's lifting with care, paying attention to your posture and ergonomics, sitting comfortably when driving, and being aware of the position of your back when doing chores or other similar jobs, as suggested in IDEAS 4, 5, and 42.

Try another idea...

So anticipate any dangerous situations. Let people back at base know where you are and when you're due back, so they can take action if you don't show up. Carry a personal attack alarm—and make sure it's in working order and constantly ready on hand. Learn how to defuse any situation that's feeling tense before it becomes a confrontation. (You might need assertiveness training for this.) But don't become aggressive however much you're goaded, or things could just escalate and get out of hand.

See if you can improve the way services are organized at work so that you're efficient and customers don't get frustrated waiting, or angry if something goes wrong. You need to know how to manage your anger to avoid blowing a gasket when provoked. If any violence is threatened or happens, analyze what has occurred afterward to see if there's anything you can do to avoid a recurrence. There should be a system to summon help if you need it, such as discreet emergency buzzers. And report any incidents to your employers or the police, to prevent them from happening again.

"I believe that one of life's greatest risks is never daring to take a risk."
OPRAH WINFREY

Defining idea...

How did it go?

Q **I know personal safety is important, and what you say is interesting. But what does it really have to do with beating back pain?**

A *If you're physically attacked, you're likely to fall awkwardly and strain your back. A thump or beating could cause you to have bruising or a twisting injury. Even the stress from a verbal attack could cause your back muscles to knot up at work or in dread of going out. Don't knock it—it's for your own good.*

Q **I work on the shop floor, so it's not really possible to cut out all risks to my back from work, is it?**

A *Obviously some jobs are more of a risk than others, but even if you take care with your normal lifting, you can still get caught if you do a repair or lifting job unexpectedly, like changing the wheel of your car or replacing a water jug. In a crisis situation you still have to take care of how you're lifting and carrying loads—so always lift properly and it will become automatic.*

48

Trick or treat?

**Paralyzed by the choice of treatments offered for your
back pain? Well, you could be if you don't watch out.**

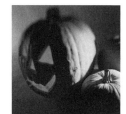

So many choices to treat your back pain,
but which is right for you? Some
treatments promoted to help back pain don't
work, or are too risky and shouldn't be tried.

DON'T LET YOURSELF BE MANIPULATED

Being manipulated under general anesthetic may cause serious neurological
damage. With you lying there completely relaxed and floppy, your muscles and
ligaments will put up little resistance to the practitioner exerting potentially
damaging movements on the vertebrae of your spine. The problem is, you're not
a rag doll, even if you look like one. Sharp thrusts on the vertebrae can cause
bones to compress or shatter nerves running through them as they emerge from
the spinal canal. You could be paralyzed as a result or get persisting muscle
weakness.

Here's an idea for you...

It may seem basic, but before being manipulated, check that you're being treated by a reputable practitioner who's been properly trained. Look up their qualifications on the website of their professional body. Before treating you they should learn all about you, your symptoms, and your past medical history. This, coupled with their professional acumen and examination, should minimize the chance of them not picking up on other serious conditions before they manipulate your spine.

DON'T WEAR A BODY BRACE

Wearing a body brace around a painful back may give you sores from where it rubs against your skin, and it could encourage your spine to stiffen up and lead to your trunk muscles wasting. It can be difficult to breathe when you've got such a tight band around you, too.

AVOID CERTAIN DRUGS

Steroid drugs may relieve the inflammation causing your back pain to some extent, but will have complications if you use them for longer than the short term. Possible complications are a stomach ulcer, where you risk a bleed; weight gain around your trunk and face; thinning of your skin; and an increased likelihood of developing diabetes and blood pressure problems. Anti-inflammatory drugs can also provoke a stomach ulcer in susceptible people.

Muscle relaxants such as diazepam can relieve painful muscle spasms, but beware of these as you may easily become addicted. They can also make you drowsy, and that could have repercussions if you nod off while driving a car or operating machinery. Strong painkillers can make you feel drowsy, too, and may have other side effects, like constipation or hallucinations. Some people become dependent on the codeine-containing drugs they take for pain relief, which is even more likely with morphine-based medication.

GOING WRONG WITH COMPLEMENTARY THERAPIES

Some of the hands-on complementary therapies can be quite forceful. If you have cancer or infection in the bones of your spine, or osteoporosis causing thinning of your bones, then you might get a fracture in one of your vertebrae from over-energetic manipulation.

So long as acupuncture is undertaken by a trained professional, you'll be fine. But if you get some Jones-the-Needle from the backstreets who doesn't use disposable needles or has inadequate sterilization procedures, you could be laying yourself open to infection. Why risk getting hepatitis or HIV from a dirty needle for the sake of a few pennies?

SAY NO TO X-RAYS ON YOUR BACK

The excessive radiation involved in spinal X-rays is very dangerous, for what is usually very little, or no, useful diagnostic information. If you go to a doctor and nag her to X-ray your back, you might get it done. But when she puts the film on the light box and shows you a blurry image, you'll only see what a fool you've been.

Take care with herbal medicines. **IDEA 22, *Find your roots*, will tell you that just because they're natural doesn't mean that they're harmless.**

Try another idea...

"Knowledge is power."
ANONYMOUS

Defining idea...

ALLERGIC TO OILS?

You might be allergic to one or more of the aromatherapy oils. If so, you'll come out in a very itchy rash that may last for one or more days. Some people think that some aromatic oils have the potential to cause cancer (but then, some people think golf is a sport).

DON'T BURN

Don't hold an ice pack on the same area of the skin for more than 10 minutes or you'll risk getting an ice burn. This will kill that area of the skin so that it sloughs off, leaving you with a raw area. Overdoing a heat pack on bare skin will do pretty much the same thing.

Q   **Are any of the back treatments especially dangerous for me, now that I'm expecting?**

How did it go?

A   *If you're pregnant you'll need to be particularly careful of many of the treatments available for back pain. Acupuncture, for instance, could inadvertently use needle sites that serve a dual purpose and risk stimulating labor. Manipulation would be difficult, as you'd be unable to lie comfortably on your stomach and take pressure on your spine. The wrong herbal medicines could be harmful to the baby. You won't want to take painkillers, even if they're prescribed by a doctor (you might be begging for them come the time; but don't worry about that now). Pilates exercises are okay after the first 14 weeks of pregnancy, but as with any exercises, you have to be careful not to over-exert yourself.*

Q   **Everything sounds risky, so I think I'll just lie here on the couch until I'm better. Nothing wrong with that, is there?**

A   *Years ago, people with back pain were encouraged to rest in bed. But we now know that that's bad advice. Your back will just stiffen up and your muscles will grow weaker through disuse. You might also get pressure sores and be more likely to develop a blood clot, which could cause a heart attack, pulmonary embolism, or stroke. So best to get up and about as soon as you can.*

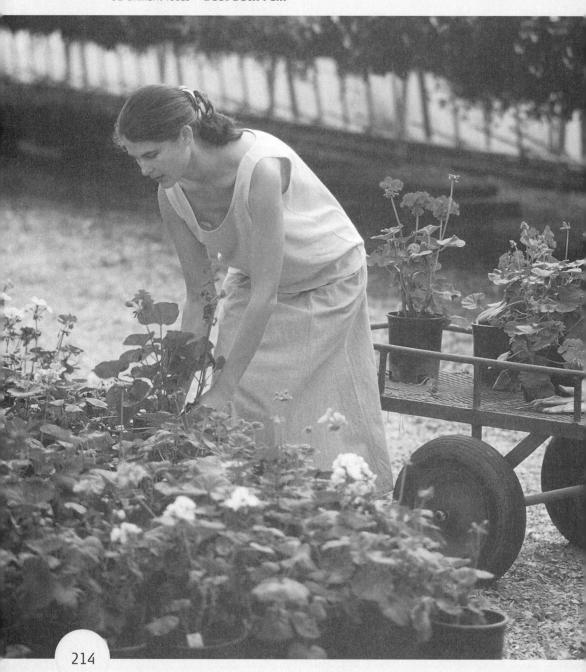

49

Out of work

The best hobbies are interesting yet restful, cost little and even generate money, keep you fit but don't wear you out or strain your back. If your hobby doesn't match up, enjoy it anyway!

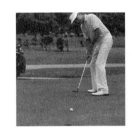

Preserving your back should be your hobby horse. Always make sure you enjoy the ride.

If you've had back pain for a while, maybe one of your hobbies could be triggering the problem. If so, don't just give it up—try finding another way of doing it that doesn't put your back under such strain. If you've got a competitive hobby or sport, or are just a competitive person by nature, then it could be that you're stressing your back muscles when you get worked up about winning (or not). If that's you, relax—take the pressure off. You'll probably perform better that way anyway.

STANDING AROUND

Some hobbies will mean you standing around for hours on end. Maybe it's watching football or another sport, or it could be that shopping is your retail therapy. Is it worth the discomfort afterward? Could you sit down instead of standing for so long? You could buy more of your clothes or other stuff from catalogs, when sitting at home, and just go to the stores for special purchases or when you really know what you want.

See if there's something else you can do to avoid bending over. Check if you need new glasses, so you can hold your head farther away from what you're doing. Get a magnifying glass or sheet so that you can sit farther back from your handiwork. Switch to a different aspect of the same hobby that doesn't require such close work. If you're set on sewing, opt for lightweight materials that'll suit your back.

Would watching the match on a wide-screen TV with lots of others, as in a bar, be a substitute for standing at the side of the field? You'd still be in the thick of the crowd. If you do have to stand still, then do some of the exercises that you've learned from the complementary practitioners to keep your back and abdominal muscles moving.

The ultimate in standing around is to be employed as an artistic statue, holding mimes or frozen positions to entertain the crowds. Don't do it—the money's lousy anyway.

SITTING AROUND

You can spend ages stooping over a workbench or table with some hobbies, like stamp collecting or embroidery. If you're entranced by what you're doing, you may not notice how much your neck and back ache until it's too late and you've overstrained both. It's important that you don't forget to take regular breaks to walk around and stretch, so set an alarm clock to remind you, or get someone to check in on you.

CUT THE RISK FROM YOUR HOBBY

Some contact sports will inevitably put your back at risk. With football or rugby, it's common for players to get hurt from a tackle. You need to find a sport where you're more in control of your movements rather than one where you're likely to twist your back muscles or jar your spine in collisions with other people.

Some hobbies are going to give you a bumpy ride that could jar your back, like horse riding or off-road racing with bikes or cars. When you come down to earth with a bump you don't want it to be with a painful back. Switch to watching horse racing or running veteran cars—develop a related but safer hobby.

Learn to be more aware of your body through yoga or Pilates— see IDEA 14, *Strike a pose*, and IDEA 20, *At the core of the matter*.

Try another idea...

Your hobby might seem safe but have hidden dangers. You might be into antiques and not realize the amount of lifting involved at antiques fairs, transporting your goods, setting up and dismantling stalls. There may be no one around to help you lift that solid mahogany table or gigantic grandfather clock. As a stamp collector you might have overlooked the overnight travel involved in attending stamp fairs across the country. All those strange beds, in cheap hotels with rickety furniture, may save your money for your stamps, but at what price?

Then there's breeding animals—can there be dangers here? Well, yes. If you're breeding any pets—parrots or goats, for instance—you'll probably need to be up through the night feeding them when they're young. And your back may suffer if you don't get a full night's rest. There'll be a lot of clearing up after them, and you may even have to dodge a kick or two as they grow bigger (that's the goat, not the parrot).

"Every day brings a chance for you to draw in a breath, kick off your shoes, and dance."
OPRAH WINFREY

Defining idea...

217

How did it go?

Q I think I'd better settle for something less energetic, like becoming a movie buff or regular theatergoer. They're safe, surely?

A *Well, safe-ish. You're not going to be sawn in half, but you might have to do some endurance sitting. If you like going to the movies or theater, make the most of any breaks in the program—blockbusters may mean sitting there for three hours at a time. Make an excuse and go to buy a drink midway through, so you can stretch. Don't forget to take your lumbar roll with you so you can sit more comfortably.*

Q My friends are planning to go on an adventure vacation in the Caribbean and I'm not sure whether to risk going with them. Do you think I should play it safe?

A *Weigh the thrill you get from dangerous hobbies like hang-gliding or parachuting with the risk of hurting your back as you take your weight or land awkwardly on the ground. Find out as much as possible about the likely risks and how much you'll pay to do that bungee jump, parachute drop, or whatever safely. Ask the company booking the adventure parts of the trip about safety measures, and check that your travel insurance covers you for dangerous sports in case there's an accident and you need professional help.*

50

Living as a different you

Ready, set, go. That can still be your motto after hurting your back, though get ready to walk rather than race through life. The key word is "go," not "stay" or "sit."

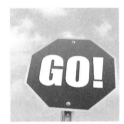

Think of what you can do rather than what you can do no longer...and then do it.

DON'T GIVE UP

So you've had an accident and hurt your back. Maybe you've fallen over and twisted it. You may have been a driver or passenger in a car crash, or been bumped from behind while your car was stationary. Maybe you've had a whiplash injury to your neck and your back hurts, too. You might have had an operation on your back that hasn't been as successful as hoped. Whatever—you're now walking with a cane or sitting in a wheelchair because of your back pain or injury.

That's tough. But the key thing is not to give up trying to improve the quality of your life. That might be trying to walk again, with or without a stick, or minimizing your pain. Don't let other people make you an invalid by doing everything for you. Keep doing whatever you can for yourself so that you're as independent as possible, even if your back hurts. Don't be ridiculous, though, and try to do something that can only make you worse.

Here's an idea for you... **Just because you are no longer able doesn't mean that you have to give up your hobby. Instead, adapt the way you do it. If you usually play sport, then go and watch it instead. If you were into sailing or boats, find a disabled sailing club where others will help you sail as you did before, or see if local able-bodied clubs can make special arrangements.**

INSIST ON KNOWING WHAT TO DO

Act on the advice from the health practitioners looking after you. If your physical therapist tells you to exercise regularly, do it. Don't put off doing exercises just because they hurt. Take some painkillers an hour or so before you intend to do the exercises, so that it's easier to do them for longer.

There may be a delay between getting therapy started when you come home from the hospital, so ask the hospital therapists what to do when you get home and seek advice about exercise, washing, dressing, sleeping, and the like. Keep calling and making a nuisance of yourself until you get all the advice and help you need from the health professionals. Make sure you're clear on how much weight you can bear on your legs if you're walking with crutches or a cane.

BE AS INDEPENDENT AS POSSIBLE

Organize your house so that you can be as
independent as possible. If you're going to be
in a wheelchair for a while, buy or get someone
to make a ramp for your front or back door so
you can wheel yourself in and out whenever
you want to. Set up your bed on the ground
floor if stairs are a problem. That way, you'll
stay in the midst of things and not languish in your sickbed out of sight—and out
of mind. Get a bath or shower seat so that you can wash and bathe as often as you
used to. Borrow or buy an ejector chair so that you can get up and down without
help or pulling too much on your back. With one of these, you can even transfer to
a wheelchair unaided.

Go to a gym and book an appointment with a personal trainer. They'll know the
best type of exercise machines for you. If you're off work with your back problem
and therefore able to go when it's quiet, you could get the added bonus of a bargain
deal for off-peak use of the gym or pool.

FIND A NEW HOBBY

Make the most of the extra time on your hands if you're unavoidably out of work or
unable to go out on the town or socialize. Learn a new skill like photography, or do
a university-based distance learning course and
get a new qualification. If you can manage
something like that it will give you some
excitement and help you to develop yourself.

Try another idea...

Ask your partner to massage
your back and other parts of
your body that are tense or
painful. They could massage
aromatic oils into your painful
areas and really help your
muscles relax—look at IDEA 15,
Ahead by a nose.

*"I want to be all that I am
capable of becoming..."*
KATHERINE MANSFIELD

Defining idea...

221

How did it go?

Q **I want to get back to work after my back injury, but I'm not sure if I can do the lifting part of the job I did before. What should I do?**

A *If your work has an occupational health department or can get advice, they can assess your disability and organize for you to work in a different capacity, or they could provide equipment to help you do your work despite your health problems. They should also be able to give you expert advice about doing things in different ways. There may be a government fund that could pay for adaptations in your workplace.*

Q **I'm sick of being left at home in my wheelchair when the rest of my family flies off for a break because I'm too nervous to venture far. What do you advise?**

A *There's lots of help to get you on trains and planes—just call ahead and inquire. Ask about arranging help when you make your booking. Some vacation companies specialize in arranging vacations for people with disabilities. In Mexico, for instance, you can even hire a wheelchair with big wheels so you can get around on the sand at the beach. I don't think they've invented wheelchair beach volleyball yet, but I'm sure it's only a matter of time.*

51

Occupational hazards

Things just aren't what they used to be—thank goodness. Now we've got hydraulic lifts, legislation, and gadgets to protect our backs—most of the time.

Some jobs are riddled with unexpected hazards. But the most risky thing is if you forget to be sensible and take a chance doing an awkward lift.

TYPE OF WORK

People working in retail, food service, construction, water, and health service sectors, as well as in mining and agriculture, are most likely to suffer from back pain. About one-third of people in professional and skilled non-manual occupations complain of back pain, compared with half of those in manual and unskilled jobs.

HOLY ORDERS

That's the priest kind, not the ordering of pizza by the armchair god in front of the TV. You might think that a priest has a back-easy life, but what about the getting down on their knees to pray, carrying heavy boxes of bric-a-brac to and from the church fair, and

Here's an idea for you... **If you're in a job where your work means you bend over for long periods, give yourself frequent breaks. Stretch and move about every 15–30 minutes or so. The amount of strain on your back will depend on how heavy the job is, so you may need to stand up and rotate your muscles even more often.**

the general stress of a 24-hour working day? For a priest, being all things to all men might include mowing the grass in the churchyard, do-it-yourself repairs around the church, and clearing up after parish meetings.

YOU WOOD DO IT

Carpenters often get back pain. There are heavy objects to lift and awkward positions to work in. You might be tempted to stretch too far over a bench to trim some wood. If you're operating a jigsaw or portable power tool, keep your back straight and don't get distracted by the job in hand.

TEACHERS

Teachers have to carry books or heavy piles of kids' classwork to grade. There'll be occasions when a child is naughty or someone faints, when suddenly you're involved in some fracas and you may hurt your back by getting into an awkward position. Keep moving and don't stand still in front of the class for long periods. And then there's the stress of the job and all that muscle tension for you to beat.

WORKING IN CONSTRUCTION

Any type of job that involves repair work is going to involve squatting, bending, and carrying loads, whether it's in major building construction or more limited home tasks. An electrician, plumber, or builder will be working at varying heights, in cramped environments and to deadlines that will tempt them to rush and forget about preserving their backs.

CLEANERS ARE A FORGOTTEN RACE

We drop trash at work or in the street without thinking of others who come after us, cleaning up the mess. Use all the mechanical help you can get. If there's better equipment for cleaning floors, petition the boss for it. If a cleaning cloth or fluid would mean less elbow grease, get hold of it. Use a feather duster on a long pole so you don't have to stretch so far. Carry several loads of reasonable weight rather than one or two over-heavy ones—less water in the buckets, lighter bags of trash.

Use equipment to help with lifting and don't chance lifting loads over the limits recommended in IDEA 6, *Ooh, you don't want to do that...*

Try another idea...

COOKS

Cooks lift heavy pans full of vegetables in water, huge meat dishes, and heavy puddings. That lifting can be your downfall, especially if you twist your trunk to shift heavy pans from one burner to another rather than move your feet, or if the cooking surface is too high to be a comfortable lift. Don't do it. Cook in smaller quantities so that the lifting is easier. And if a chef gets hysterical over meeting customers' orders, don't let it get your back tense.

DRIVING YOU CRAZY

If you're a long-distance truck driver or company rep, you're on the road for long periods. The vibration of the truck's engine can jigger up your spine, wearing your discs. Then there's all that clambering around on the loads to tie them on safely and unloading the

"A human being must have occupation if he or she is not to become a nuisance to others."
DOROTHY L. SAYERS

Defining idea...

delivery at the other end. As a truck driver you'll doubtless be sleeping in your truck to save money on overnight accommodation. As a company rep you'll be stuck in a car that's not specially designed for all-day driving, though the sound system will be pretty good.

POLICE AND FIRE SERVICE

If you work for the police or fire service, you might be carrying or dragging people out of danger (or cats out of trees) or shifting heavy equipment. You'll be vulnerable to attack by drunks or violent thugs. As a police officer, you might diversify in your career—handling dogs, working underwater, riding horses, sitting at a computer for a long time, or highway driving. As a fire officer there'll be heavy breathing apparatus and lots of practice for unpredictable situations—climbing ladders, crawling in smoke-filled rooms, carrying dummies to safety.

Q **What's the safest occupation for not straining my back further?**

How did it go?

A *Sleeping policeman springs to mind, but then there's all the cars to contend with... Most jobs involve some lifting or bending over, even if it's not obvious from the job description. Go for an occupation where you move around a lot, sometimes sitting, sometimes walking. With office work check that you can vary the type of tasks you do and get out of the office occasionally. If it's heavy work, is there lifting equipment and is the boss sensible?*

Q **I'm out of work with a bad back. I figure that it was work that caused it, so if I go back it will only get worse. Should I just give up and stay at home?**

A *No—get back to work as soon as you can. It's best to keep moving. See if you can do a light job, or work from home for a while. If you do everything by the book, you shouldn't harm yourself further. And being occupied and returning to something of a normal life will help your recovery.*

227

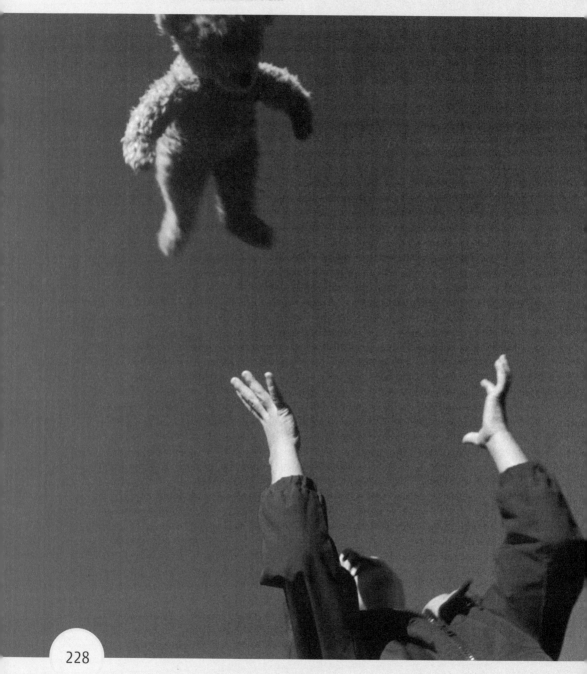

52

Nothing is beyond your reach

Information is power. If you've got it, flaunt it. Then the therapists or doctors you consult should treat you well and won't brush you off with big words.

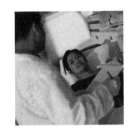

Do your homework and study up on treatments for back pain on the Internet. Or go down to the local library and see what information they've got there.

What you want to know will depend on your diagnosis and how well the practitioners treating you have explained what's wrong. You'll probably want information about how to prevent or relieve your pain, what treatment options are available to you, and their relative risks and benefits.

Here's an
idea for
you... **Websites can give you relevant information you never even realized existed. If you type in "back pain" or other general term using a common search engine you'll be inundated by thousands of hits. But beware— not all information is reliable. Check the provenance before deciding the providence.**

READ ALL ABOUT IT

Educational leaflets and books are great for giving you more information in a general way. Hopefully they're written in simple, clear language, so you're not more confused than before you started reading them. You'll want information that applies to you, your body size and shape, your circumstances, your occupation, or your diagnosis.

If you still want more, go intellectual. If you want to do it right you could search an electronic database that covers medical and nursing fields. Some include reviews of the reputable research published on the subject you're interested in. That's a good place to start, for it means that experts have made a judgment about what the key research means. Go to your nearest health library and you'll be able to access these sorts of reviews, or take a subscription out from home (for example, www.clinicalevidence.com).

DO A SEARCH OF THE ORIGINAL LITERATURE YOURSELF

Here's how to do it: Although you may be burning to ask your question, when you try to set it down on paper you may find that it's more difficult than you think. Questions have to be phrased in a very specific way to obtain meaningful responses. The question you want to answer from searching the Internet should be simple and specific. For instance, it could be "What are the risks from spinal surgery?" rather than "What's the best treatment for back pain?" Focus and phrase your question to include whatever it is that you want to know about effects or efficiency of treatments, diagnosis, or outlook for you.

How long you spend and to what lengths you go with a search of the Internet will depend on its purpose. Write down the keywords you want to use and prioritize their order of importance. How many keywords you enter at the first stage depends on how wide you expect your field of inquiry to be. If you type in "back pain" you will get thousands more references to published research than if you type in a rare condition, like "ankylosing spondylitis."

Try the Medline database produced by the National Library of Medicine. You can access it without a password via the PubMed website (www.ncbi.nlm.nih.gov/PubMed/medline.html). It has a phenomenal number of references, so use a very strict search strategy to narrow down your focus of inquiry. Search for the keyword(s) you've chosen in the title or abstract of any published research. Limit your search by combining keywords using the instructions "and" and "or." Then read the research papers (or their abstracts) you identify in your search.

Chat to others and hear about their experiences of complementary medicine and conventional treatments as in IDEA 45, *Listening in.*

Try another idea...

"Be careful about reading books. You may die of a misprint."
MARK TWAIN

Defining idea...

After all this, you'll be far better informed next time you go to see a doctor or therapist. In fact, you may well know more about the reliability and risks of alternative treatments than they do! Don't show off or show them up—they'll become defensive and you may lose their goodwill in helping you to get better.

CONTACT SELF-HELP ORGANIZATIONS OR PROFESSIONAL BODIES

They'll send you information or advice about their special fields. But even if their information is accurate, it may not give you the whole picture, as they may be disseminating biased information that shows their work in a good light.

How did **Q Are there any good websites to get more information about**
it go? **treatments for back pain, and how I can do my utmost to care for**
my back?

A *Here's a selection:*

www.webmd.com
www.spine-health.com
www.back.com (has videos of exercises and spinal surgery)
www.bbc.co.uk/health/backchat
http://familydoctor.org/x2563.xml
www.nlm.nih.gov/medlineplus/backpain.html
www.self-realization.com/yoga_directory.htm

Q **Can you help me find out more about various alternative medicines from professional organizations across the world? Will they provide more reliable information?**

A *You could look at the websites given above, as well as those of the professional bodies below. Different countries give different guidance, so you're better off checking out anything you find on the Internet against research reported via the Medline database and the perspectives of your own doctor or therapist.*

British Acupuncture Council: www.acupuncture.org.uk
American Academy of Medical Acupuncture: www.medicalacupuncture.org
Aromatherapy Consortium: www.aromatherapy-regulation.org.uk
General Chiropractic Council: www.gcc-uk.org
American Chiropractic Association: www.amerchiro.org
National Institute of Medical Herbalists: www.nimh.org.uk
National Herbalist Association of Australia: www.nhaa.org.au
Faculty of Homeopathy: www.trusthomeopathy.org
North American Society of Homeopaths: www.homeopathy.org
British Society of Medical and Dental Hypnosis: www.bsmdh.org
Osteopathic Information Service: www.osteopathy.org.uk
Canadian College of Osteopathy: www.osteopathy-Canada.com/welcome.htm
Association of Reflexologists: www.aor.org.uk
Reflexology Association of Canada: www.reflexologycanada.ca
British Wheel of Yoga: www.bwy.org.uk

Where it's at...

52 Brilliant Ideas

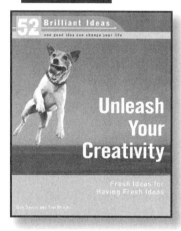

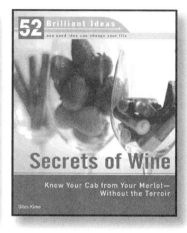

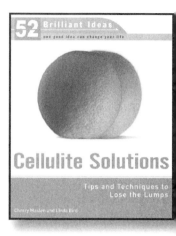

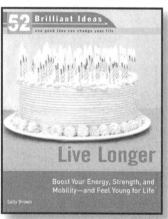

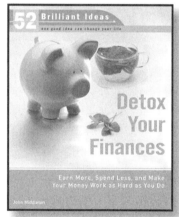

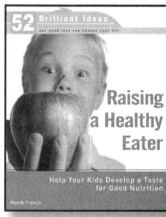

UNLEASH YOUR CREATIVITY
978-0-399-53325-9

LIVE LONGER
978-0-399-53302-0

SECRETS OF WINE
978-0-399-53348-8

DETOX YOUR FINANCES
978-0-399-53301-3

CELLULITE SOLUTIONS
978-0-399-53326-6

RAISING A HEALTHY EATER
978-0-399-53339-6

 An imprint of Penguin Group (USA)

PERIGEE

one good idea can change your life

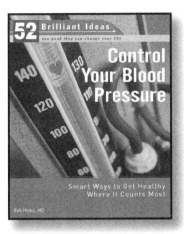
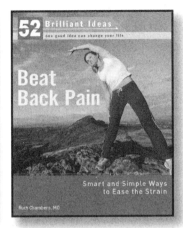
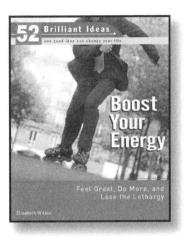
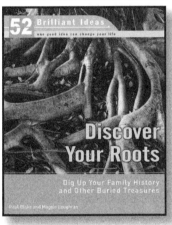
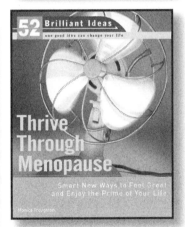
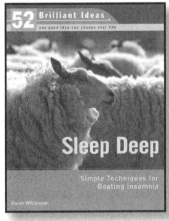